Clinical Electrocardiography
A Self-Study Course

Explanation of the cover illustrations

Original Cambridge electrocardiograph, manufactured in 1911 under agreement with Professor Willem Einthoven, the father of electrocardiography, and delivered to Dr. Thomas Lewis of the University College Hospital, London. (Photo shows Mr. Frost, the Cambridge chief inspector, acting as patient with the instrument prior to shipment to Dr. Lewis.) The second insert is of Dr. Stein, using a vector model, during a teaching session.

Historical notes

During the second half of the 19th century, the association of an electrical potential with muscular contraction was investigated by physiologists. August Waller first recorded the potential variations generated by the human heart beat in 1887 in London. In 1903 Professor Willem Einthoven completed the first electrocardiograph. He used a string galvanometer in which a very fine quartz fiber, coated with silver to make it electrically conductive and stretched between the poles of a powerful electromagnet, underwent variable displacements when the unamplified currents arising from a patient passed through it. The string was illuminated by a very bright arc lamp beam and its shadow was focused onto a moving photographic plate. A rotary spoked wheel was used to interrupt the beam at regular intervals to provide timing marks on the plate. Einthoven communicated details of his invention to Horace Darwin (later Sir Horace Darwin, F.R.S.) of the Cambridge Scientific Instrument Company in England, and to the Messrs. Edelmann in Germany, with a suggestion that they should design and manufacture, under royalty agreement, an "electrocardiograph" that could be marketed. A disagreement between Einthoven and the Edelmanns resulted in Einthoven's working exclusively with Cambridge, who manufactured their first machine in 1911 (see photo). Before 1916, 87 Cambridge electrocardiographs had been manufactured and shipped to 15 different countries as far distant as Japan, Australia, India and Russia. In 1911, Dr. Horatio B. Williams of the United States visited Einthoven and upon his return built an instrument with Charles Hindle, his mechanic. Hindle's design was good, and he established a manufacturing company, in New York State, which merged with the British firm, Cambridge Instrument Company, Ltd., in 1922, changing its name to Cambridge Instrument Company, Inc. Since then, both American and British firms have benefited from their continuing exchange of new technologies. Early on, the electrocardiograph established its value in diagnostic medicine and today maintains itself as one of the most ubiquitous electronic instruments used in modern medicine.

CLINICAL

ELECTROCARDIOGRAPHY

A SELF-STUDY COURSE

EMANUEL STEIN, M.D., M.P.H.
F.A.C.P., F.A.C.C., F.C.C.P.

Associate Dean and Director, Eastern
  Virginia Graduate School of Medicine

Professor of Internal Medicine and

Professor of Family and Community Medicine,
  Eastern Virginia Medical School,
  Norfolk, Virginia

Medical Director, United States Public
  Health Service, Ret.

Diplomate, American Board of Internal
  Medicine and Subspecialty Board of
  Cardiovascular Disease

Illustrations by
THOMAS XENAKIS, M.A., A.M.I.

Lea & Febiger   Philadelphia

Lea & Febiger
600 Washington Square
Philadelphia, Pa 19106-4198
U.S.A.
(215) 922-1330

Library of Congress Cataloging-in-Publication Data

Stein, Emanuel
    Clinical electrocardiography.

    Includes index.
    1. Electrocardiography. 2. Heart—Diseases—
Diagnosis.   I. Title.   [DNLM: 1. Electrocardiography—
problems.   WG 18 S819c]
RC683.5.E5S727   1987   616.1'207'543   86-27429
ISBN 0-8121-1088-9

PRINTED IN THE UNITED STATES OF AMERICA

Print No.   5   4

THIS WORK IS LOVINGLY DEDICATED

TO MY WIFE AND CHILDREN

for their great love, abundant
support, patience and understanding

TO MY TEACHERS

who spanned the entire experience of
electrocardiography

TO MY STUDENTS

in the classroom and in the clinic,
from whom I continue to learn

TO MY FUTURE STUDENTS

who will benefit from this effort

Preface

This book is simply written and amply illustrated to provide a firm foundation in electrocardiography for all interested members of the health professions. Some may rightfully feel that a particular subject should have been included or given more weight and that other areas have been emphasized too much. I accept full responsibility for the allocation of priorities in this synthesis of vast amounts of material. The electrocardiograms have been chosen with great care and confirmed, where possible, by clinical-pathological correlation, cardiac catheterization, X-ray and noninvasive techniques. When the question arose as to absolute accuracy versus ease of understanding in a given illustration, the decision generally was made in favor of ease of understanding. Following the adage that a picture is worth a thousand words, each illustration is carefully coordinated with the short text below it. Since a step-by-step approach is followed, it is advisable to start at the beginning and progress systematically through the book. After you have learned the basic principles of electrocardiography and have completed all the exercises and practice electrocardiograms, the book can serve as a study guide as well as a teaching, reference and review manual. As a review, the basic principles of electrocardiography can be covered in one sitting.

This method of learning to interpret electrocardiograms has been received with excitement and enthusiasm in the classroom and in the clinic. Equally exciting has been the response of patients. Throughout my years as a clinician and teacher, I have encouraged patients to take charge of their health. By utilizing this method of learning, some have followed their own progress by studying the principles of electrocardiography.

The book is divided into six chapters. The first chapter introduces the basic concepts of electrocardiography, using the vector approach. The characteristics of the normal electrocardiogram are explained and illustrated. The normal 12 lead electrocardiogram is then completely analyzed. Discussions of abnormal states, including hypertrophy, ventricular repolarization alterations, myocardial infarction, conduction disturbances and arrhythmias, comprise the remaining five chapters.

At the end of each chapter are several practice electrocardiograms related to that chapter. The analysis follows each practice electrocardiogram. At the end of the book is a series of electrocardiograms relating to all the chapters for practice and review. Here too, the analysis follows each practice electrocardiogram. It is hoped that this introduction will stimulate you to continue learning and reading electrocardiograms.

I thank Mr. R. Kenneth Bussy, Mr. Samuel Rondinelli and Ms. Dorothy DiRienzi of Lea & Febiger for their help in making this book possible, and Mr. Thomas Xenakis for elegantly translating my drawings. I should like to add my appreciation to Dr. William Fox for several electrocardiograms that have enriched this work.

Norfolk, Virginia   Emanuel Stein, M.D.

Contents

Chapter *1*

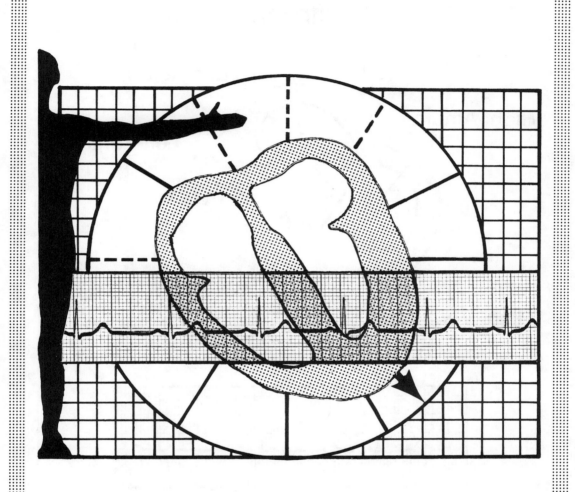

Basic Concepts and The Normal
Electrocardiogram

The Electrocardiogram

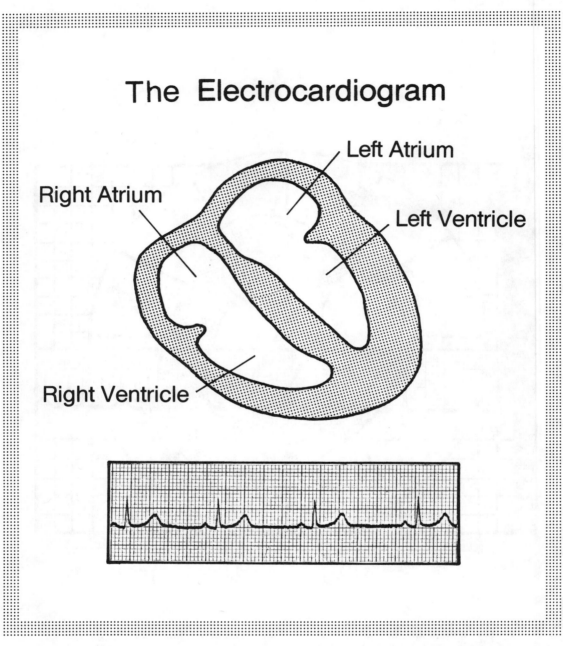

The electrocardiogram (abbreviated ECG) is a recording of the electrical activity of the heart. By the placement of electrodes on designated areas of the body, we usually record 12 views of this electrical activity. All four chambers, the left and right atria and the left and right ventricles, are represented on this recording.

1912

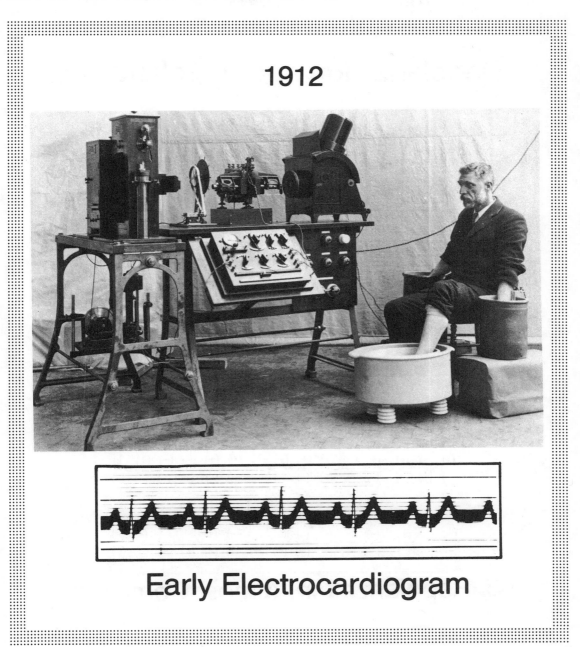

Early Electrocardiogram

It wasn't always easy to take electrocardiograms in the early days of electrocardiography. The patient had to have both arms and the left leg in containers of conducting solution (saline). The electrodes were attached to the containers, not directly to the patient. The large machine stands in sharp contrast to the compact models of today.

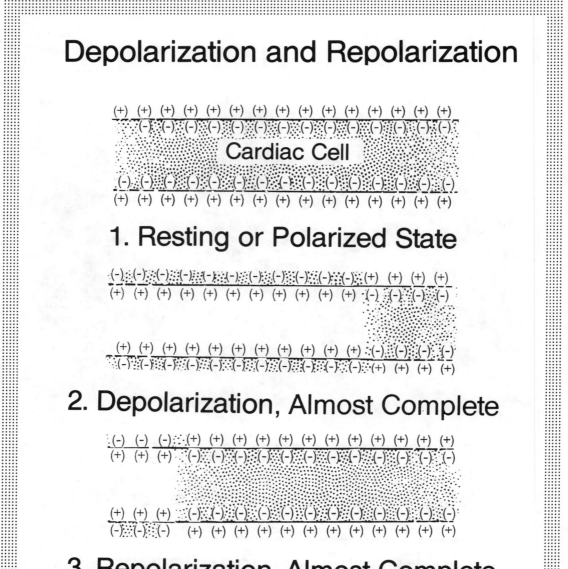

Depolarization and Repolarization

1. Resting or Polarized State

2. Depolarization, Almost Complete

3. Repolarization, Almost Complete

Depolarization and repolarization of the atria and ventricles are the *electrical* events recorded on the electrocardiogram. Depolarization is the active state and begins *before* the mechanical contraction of the respective chambers.

1. Resting or polarized state
   inside cell—negative
   outside cell—positive
2. Active state or state of depolarization
   inside cell—positive
   outside cell—negative
3. Repolarization is the restoration of the resting or polarized state.

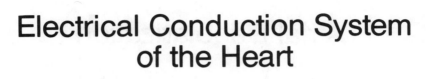

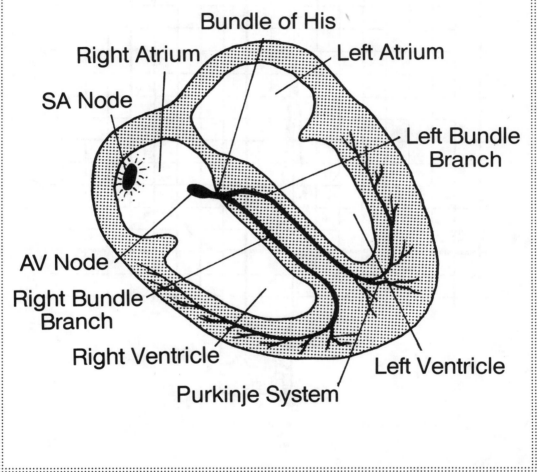

The normal site of impulse formation in the heart is the *sinoatrial (SA) node.* The atria are then depolarized. The impulse then spreads through the *atrioventricular (AV) node* and *bundle of His* to the *left (LBB) and right (RBB) bundle branches* and then to the ventricular muscle through the *Purkinje network,* leading to ventricular depolarization.

Atrial Depolarization

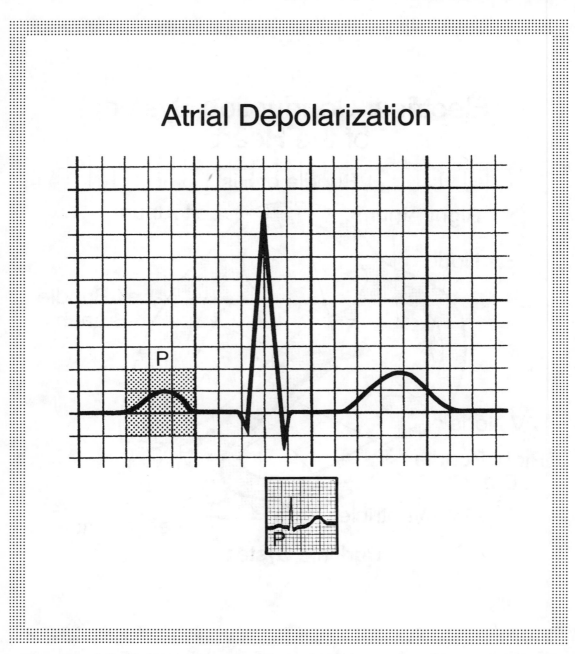

The wave of depolarization that begins in the SA node spreads to both atria, first to the right atrium, then to the left atrium. The depolarization of both atria is represented by the *P wave* on the electrocardiogram. The P wave is normally the first electrocardiographic deflection of each cardiac cycle.

PR Segment

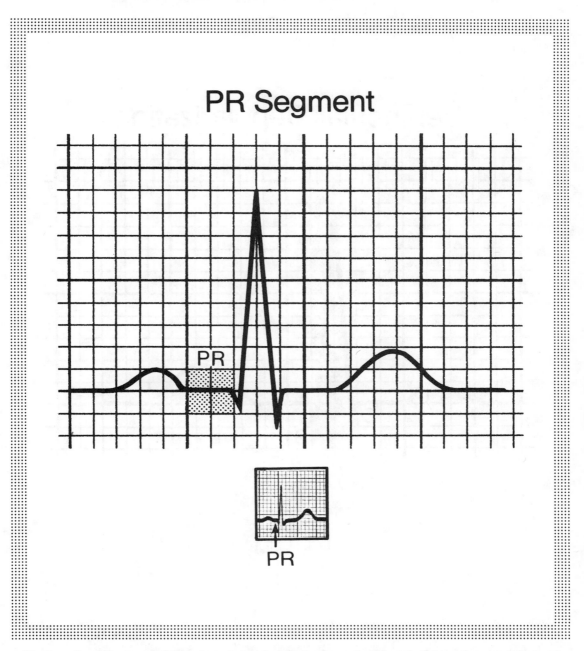

During the *PR segment*, following atrial depolarization, the electrical impulse spreads to the AV node, bundle of His and bundle branches. In the specialized electrophysiology laboratory, recordings can be made from the bundle of His using special recording techniques. On the clinical electrocardiogram, only the flat line is generally seen.

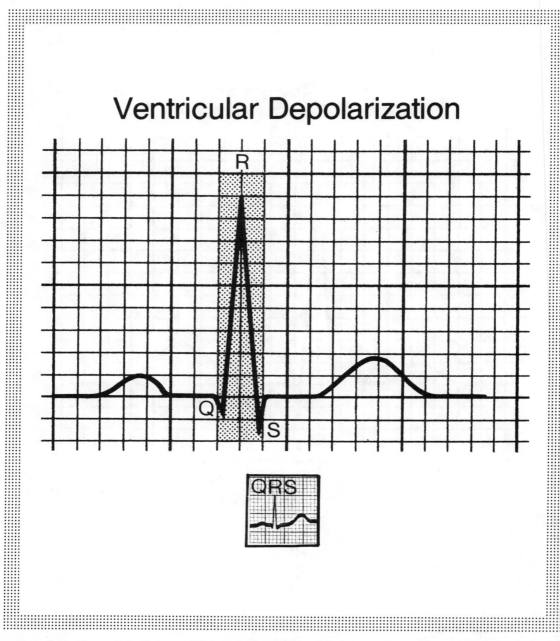

Depolarization of both ventricles is reflected in the *QRS complex.* The *R wave* is the initial positive deflection (upward, above the resting baseline of the electrocardiogram) of the QRS complex. The negative deflection (downward, inverted, occurring below the resting baseline of the electrocardiogram) *before* the R wave is the *Q wave.* The negative deflection *after* the R wave is the *S wave,* which is usually the terminal part of the QRS complex.

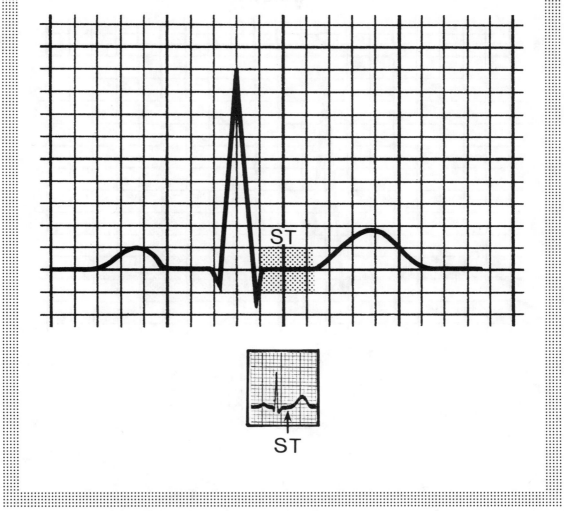

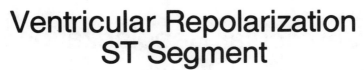

The *ST segment* extends from the end of the QRS complex to the beginning of the T wave (see next page). It represents the earlier phase of repolarization of both ventricles. The ST segment is normally isoelectric (at the same level as the resting baseline). It is neither elevated (positive) nor depressed (negative). The point at which the ST segment joins the QRS complex is known as the J (for junction) point.

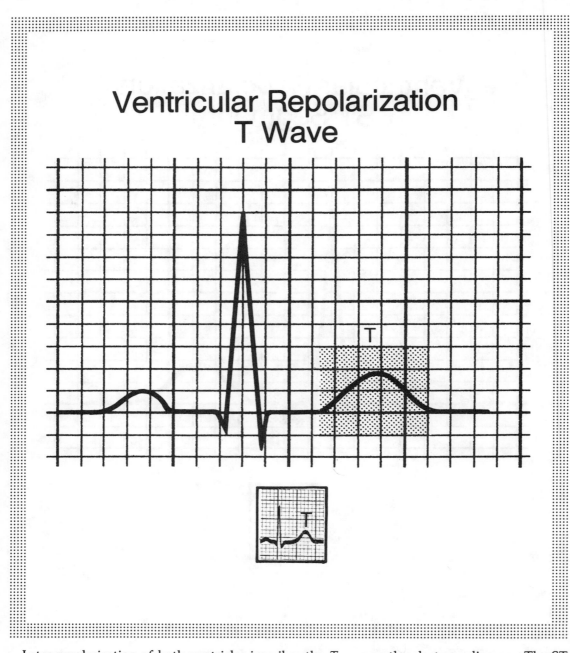

Ventricular Repolarization
T Wave

Later repolarization of both ventricles inscribes the *T wave* on the electrocardiogram. The ST segment and the T wave are sensitive indicators of the status of the ventricular myocardium.

Atrial repolarization is not often seen on the electrocardiogram because of its small size and because it coincides with the QRS complex.

Practice
Label the Electrocardiographic Waves, Intervals and Segments

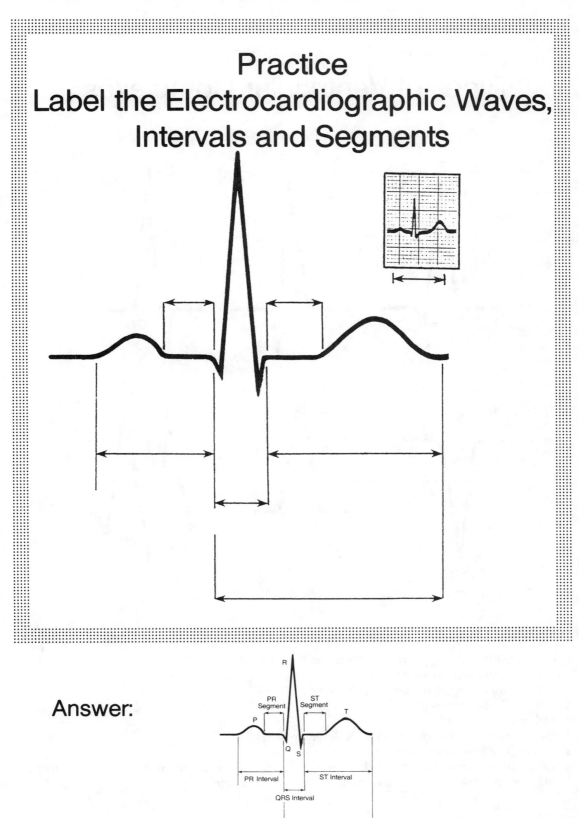

Answer:

Types of Ventricular Complexes

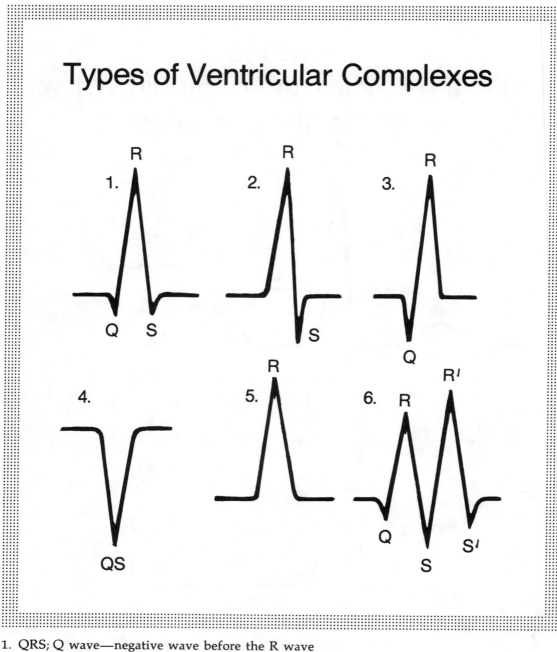

1. QRS; Q wave—negative wave before the R wave
      R wave—positive deflection
      S wave—negative after the R wave
2. RS; no Q wave present
3. QR; no S wave present
4. QS; totally negative complex, no R wave present
5. R; no Q or S waves present
6. QRSR'S', a second positive deflection after an S wave is an R' (R prime), which, in turn, may be followed by a negative deflection, an S' (S prime).

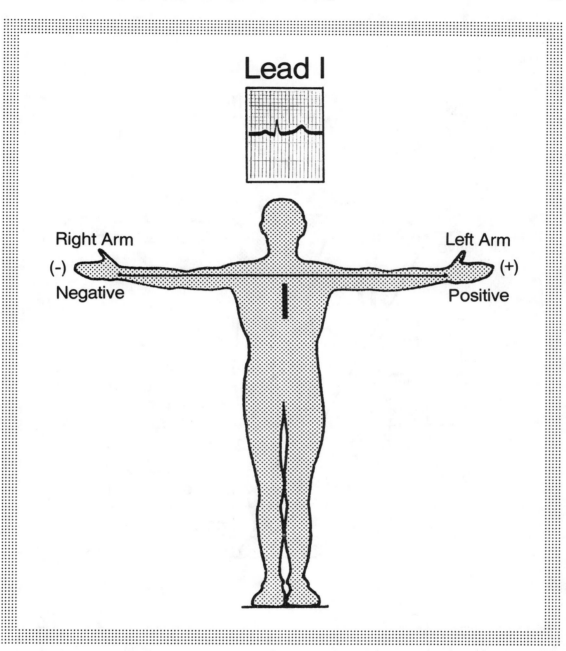

Willem Einthoven, known as the father of electrocardiography, found that by connecting the right arm to the negative electrode and the left arm to the positive electrode and inducing a current to flow, certain deflections were recorded, known as *lead I*. For recording, Einthoven used the string galvanometer, a movable writing element within a magnetic field.

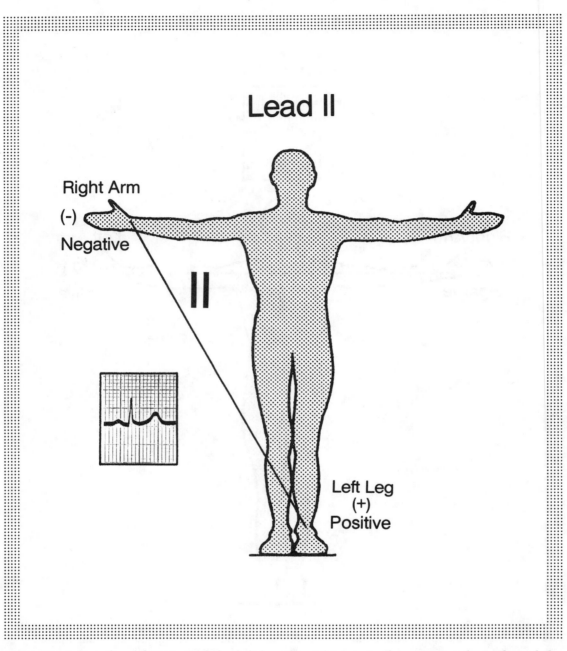

By connecting the right arm and the left leg, the right arm to the negative electrode and the left leg to the positive electrode, Einthoven recorded what became known as *lead II.*

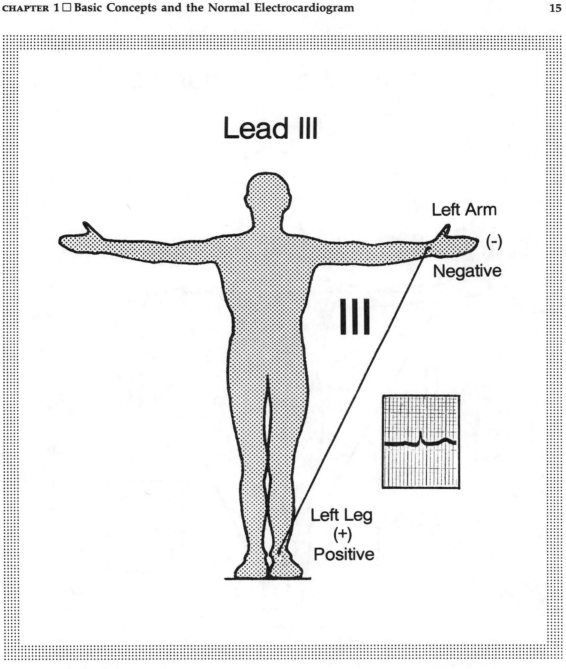

By connecting the left arm and the left leg, the left arm to the negative electrode and the left leg to the positive electrode, *lead III* is formed.

The Einthoven Triangle

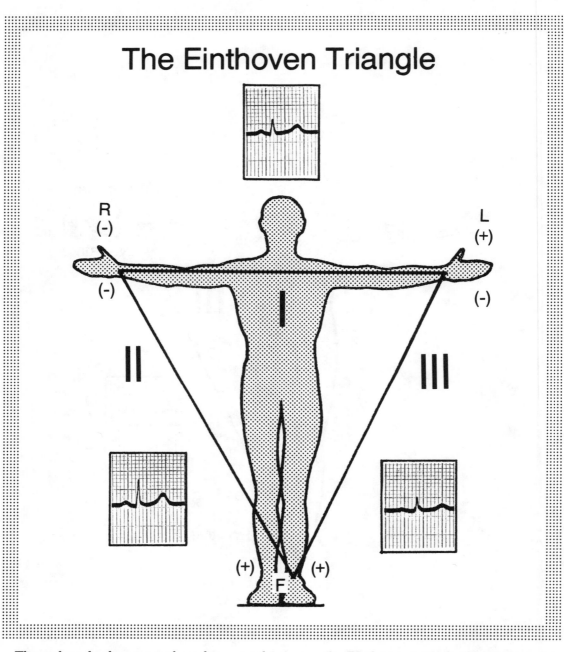

These three leads, arranged as above, are known as the Einthoven triangle. The right arm is always *negative* and the left leg is always *positive.* Note the following special relationship:

$$lead\ I\ +\ lead\ III\ =\ lead\ I\!I$$

This is an electrical truth that always holds for the *area* encompassed by each deflection. We use the heights and depths of the deflections as a good approximation. This relationship is further illustrated on the next page.

Lead I + Lead III = Lead II

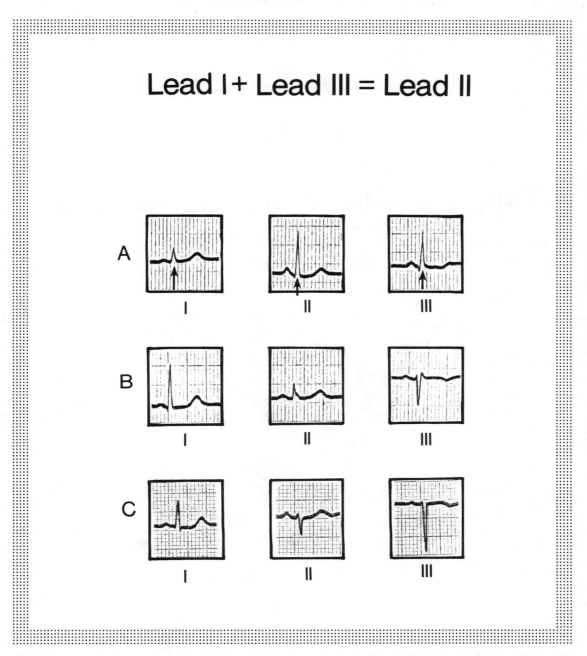

The arrows in A point to the QRS complexes in leads I, II and III. The deflection in lead I is approximately 3 mm. tall and the deflection in lead III is 9mm. tall. Using the rule that

leads I + III = lead II

the lead II deflection must be 12 mm. tall. This is true for the P as well as the T waves. Apply this relationship to B and C above.

Practice

Label the Einthoven triangle, including the polarity (+ or -) of the leads.

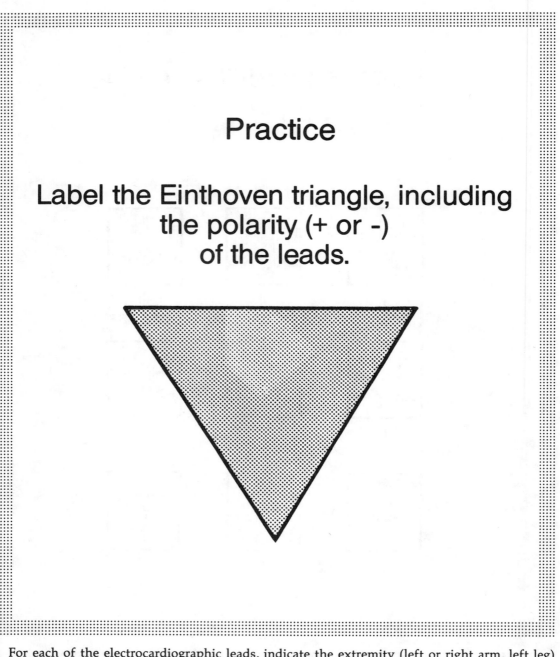

For each of the electrocardiographic leads, indicate the extremity (left or right arm, left leg) and whether it is positive (+) or negative (−).

Lead I	Lead II	Lead III
a. extremity _____	a. extremity _____	a. extremity _____
b. extremity _____	b. extremity _____	b. extremity _____

Compare with the completed Einthoven triangle on page 16.

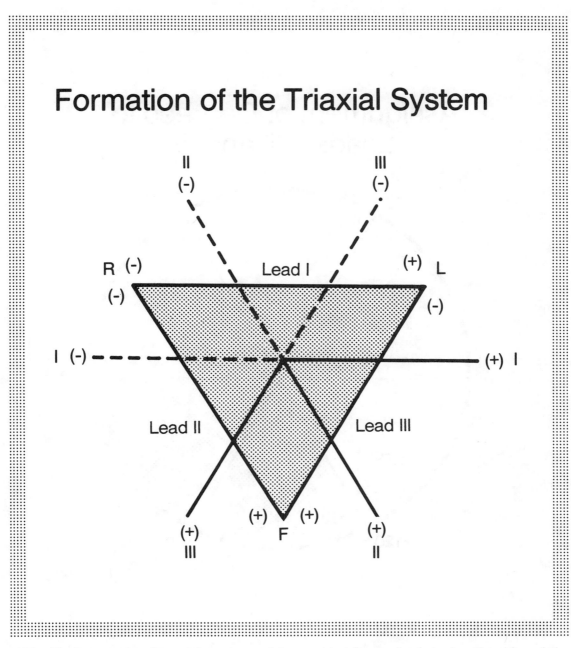

Formation of the Triaxial System

The Einthoven triangle may be converted into a *triaxial system* by bringing the sides of the triangle to the common center. The positives and negatives are now clearly delineated. The solid lines represent the positive half of each lead, whereas the broken lines represent the negative half.

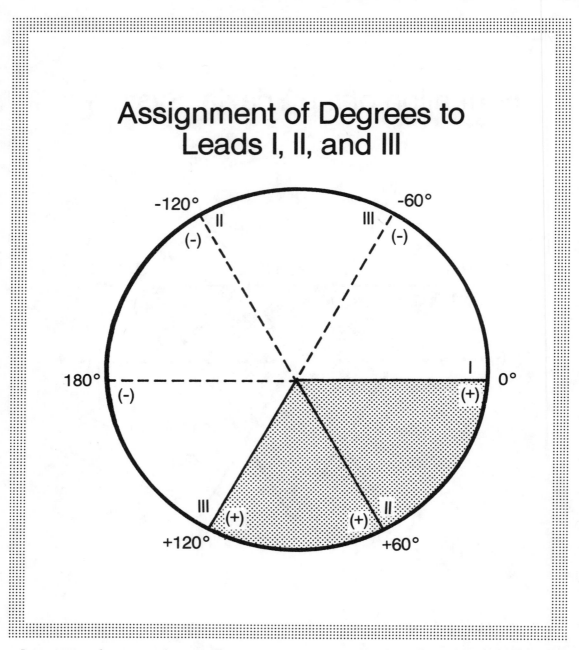

In assigning degrees to the triaxial reference system, the axes are 60° apart. The positions of the positives and negatives remain as in the Einthoven triangle.

Up to now we have been studying the three leads, I, II and III. These are the *bipolar* extremity leads; each lead makes use of two extremities. For many years these were the only leads used in electrocardiography.

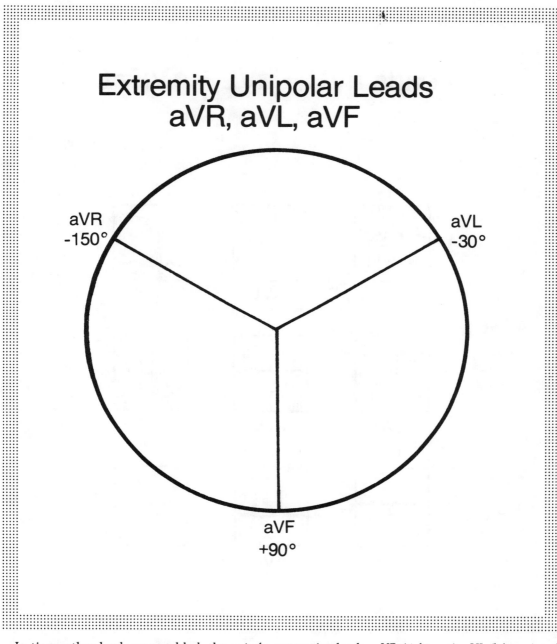

Extremity Unipolar Leads
aVR, aVL, aVF

In time, other leads were added, the *unipolar* extremity leads: *aVR (right arm), aVL (left arm)* and *aVF (left leg)*. Only one pole, the *positive,* is attached to each extremity. The negative is connected to a central terminal. The letter "a" refers to the augmentation necessary to bring these leads up to the size of leads I, II and III.

Leads aVR + aVL + aVF = 0

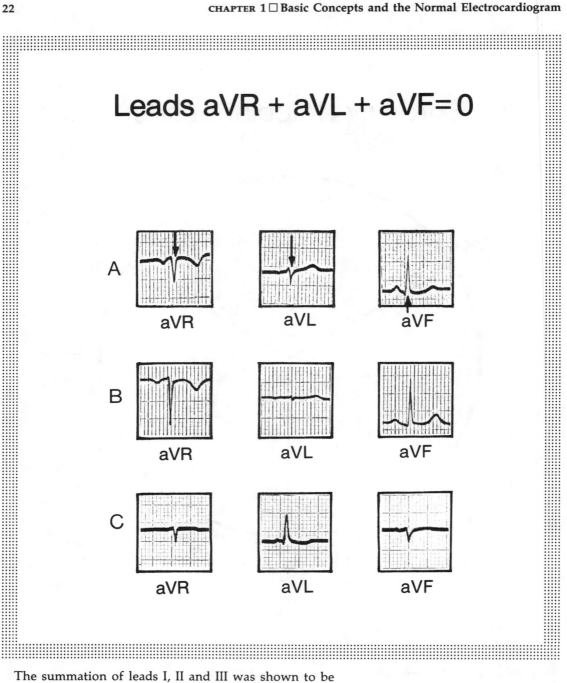

The summation of leads I, II and III was shown to be

$$lead\ I\ +\ lead\ III\ =\ lead\ II$$

The summation of leads aVR, aVL and aVF is as follows:

$$leads\ aVR\ +\ aVL\ +\ aVF\ =\ 0.$$

These relationships are of importance in the evaluation of every electrocardiogram.

Formation of Hexaxial System
I, II, III, aVR, aVL, aVF

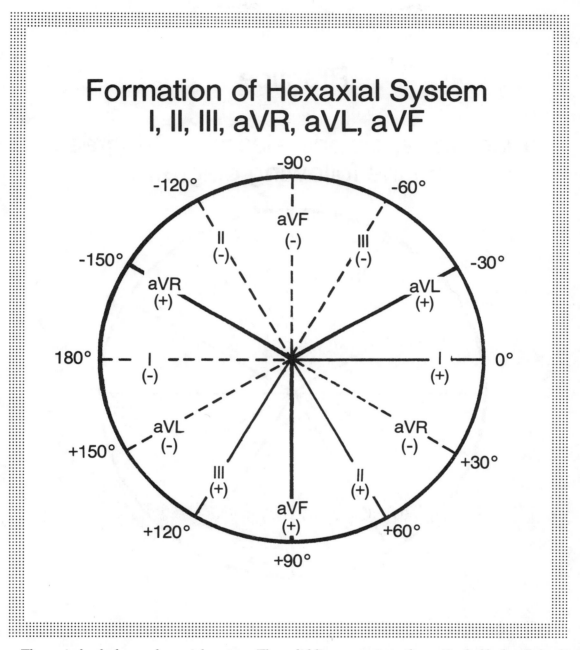

These six leads form a hexaxial system. The solid line represents the *positive* half of each lead; the broken line represents the *negative* half. The part of the circle used most frequently in clinical electrocardiography contains

positive aVL	−30°
positive I	0°
negative aVR	+30°
positive II	+60°
positive aVF	+90°
positive III	+120°

Note that *negative* aVR at +30° is used. Positive aVR is at −150°.

Practice

Place the appropriate leads and degrees on the following diagram.

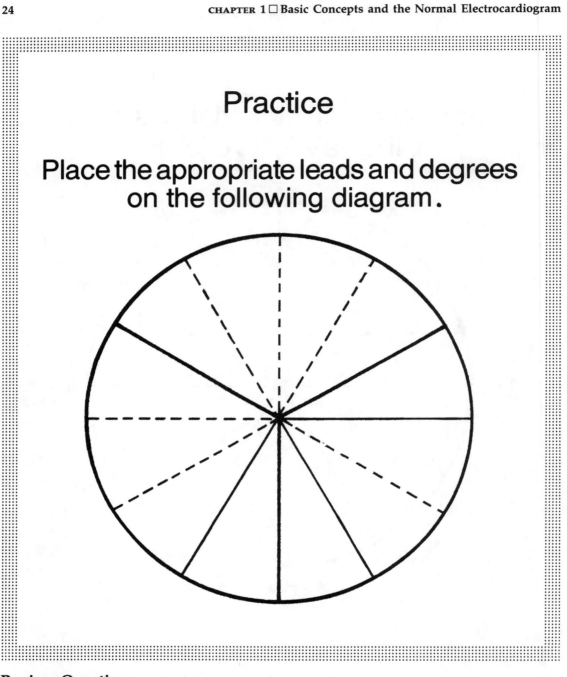

Review Questions

State the summation of leads I, II and III.

State the summation of leads aVR, aVL and aVF.

Compare with the labeled diagram on p. 23 and with the summations on p. 22.

The Cardiac Vectors

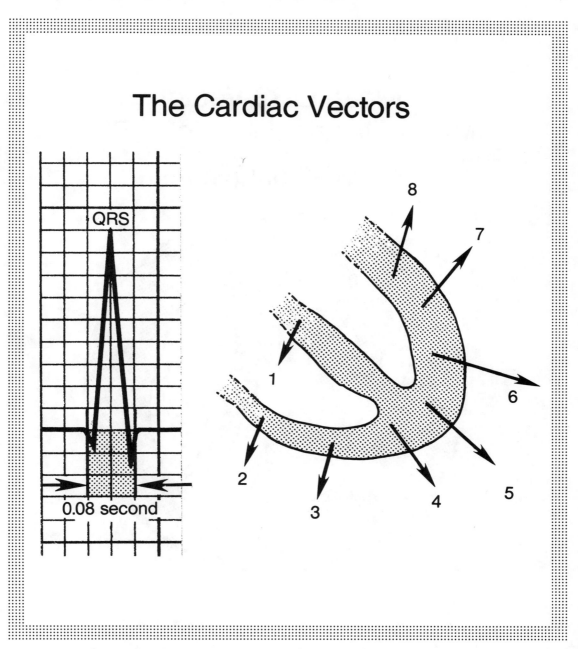

The term *vector* refers to force. In electrocardiography it refers to electrical force. A vector is represented by an arrow where both size and direction are easily demonstrated. Within a period of 0.08 sec. both ventricles are depolarized. During this single QRS interval, sequential instantaneous vectors are generated. The greater the muscle mass, the bigger the arrow will be.

Mean QRS Vector
Mean Electrical Axis of QRS
"Axis" of QRS

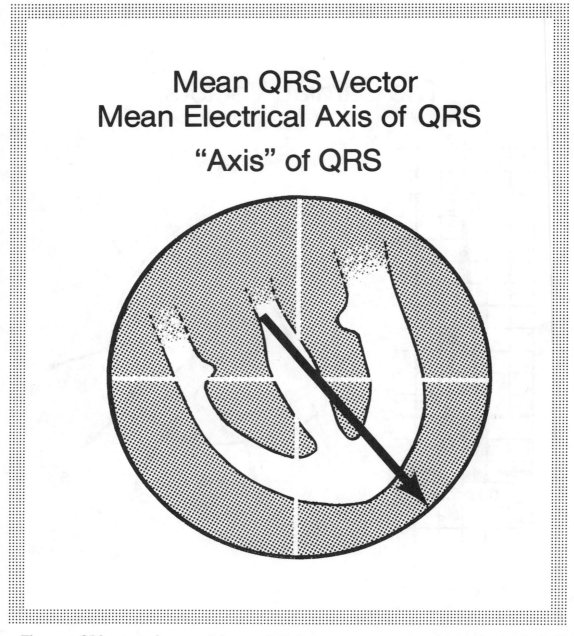

The *mean QRS vector* is the vectorial sum of all the instantaneous vectors within a single QRS interval. We often refer to the mean QRS vector, mean T vector and mean P vector in the study of electrocardiography. Because of common usage, the terms *mean electrical axis, electrical axis* or simply *"axis"* of the QRS, T and P are used.

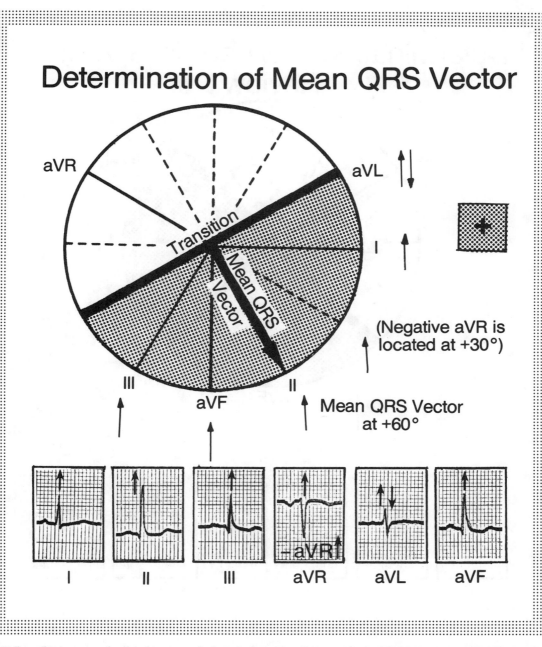

Determination of Mean QRS Vector

When lining up the leads around the circle according to their positivity or negativity, note that *negative* aVR is at +30°; lead aVR must, therefore, be inverted before being placed on the circle. Lead aVL is neither predominantly positive nor predominantly negative; the transition is therefore through lead aVL. The *mean QRS vector* is at right angles to the transitional zone on the positive side. In this electrocardiogram the *transitional zone* is at −30° and the mean QRS vector is at 60° (large arrow). The shaded area in the circle is the positive half.

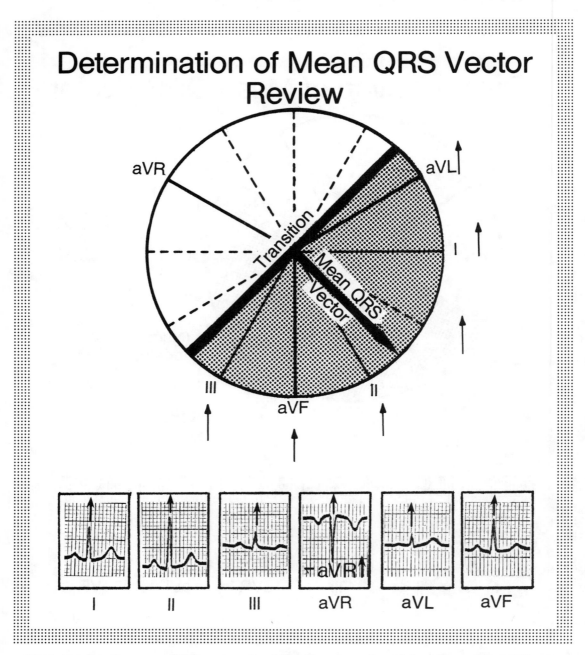

Determination of Mean QRS Vector Review

To determine the mean QRS vector, the following steps should be taken sequentially.

1. Line up all six leads on the circle according to their positivity or negativity, from −30° to +120°. Lead aVR must be inverted at +30°.
2. Draw the transition, dividing the circle into positive and negative halves.
3. The mean QRS vector is at right angles to the transition on the positive side.

In this electrocardiogram the mean QRS vector is approximately 45° (large arrow). On the next three pages, practice this determination and then check answers below.

Practice
Locate Mean QRS Vector

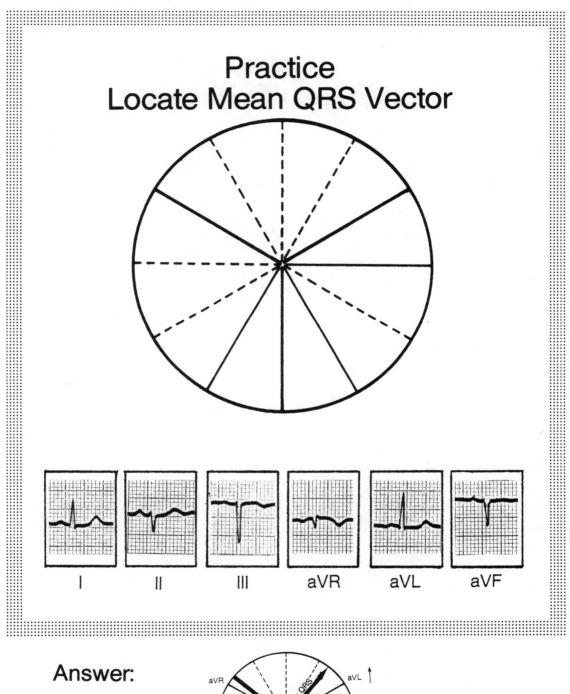

| I | II | III | aVR | aVL | aVF |

Answer:

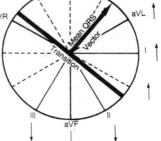

Practice
Locate Mean QRS Vector

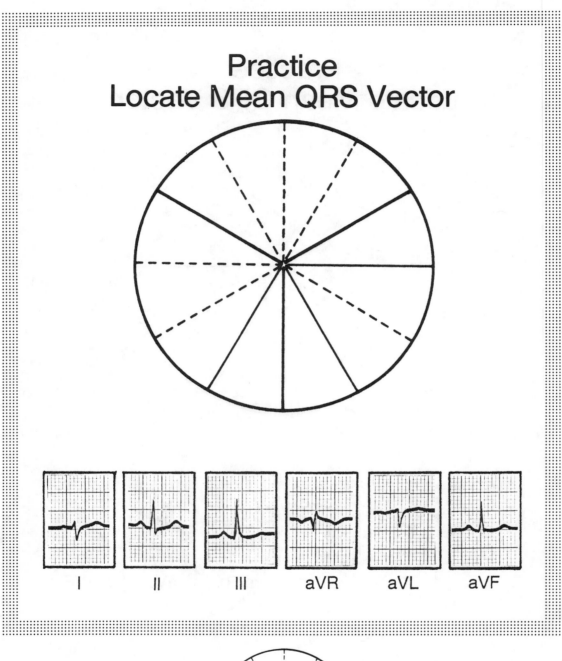

I	II	III	aVR	aVL	aVF

Answer:

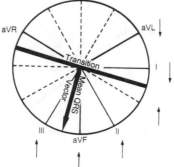

Practice
Locate Mean QRS Vector

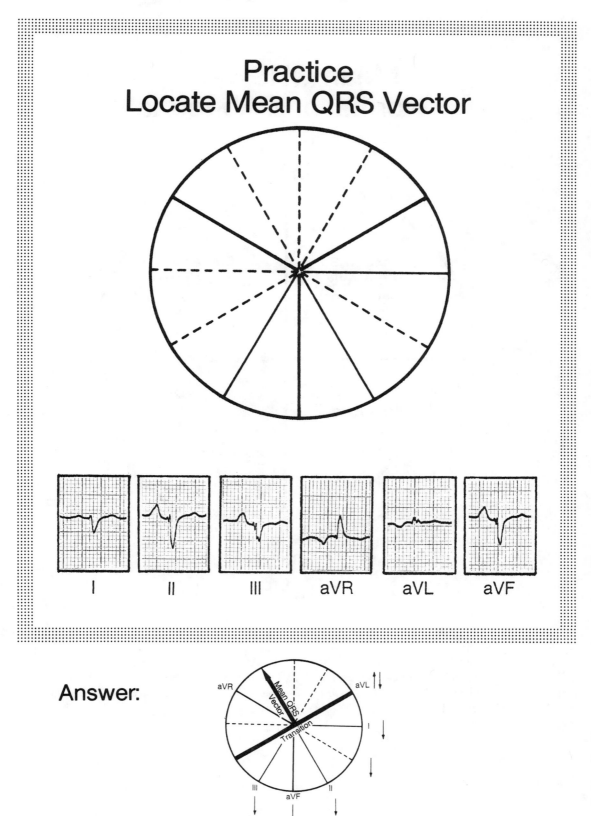

Answer:

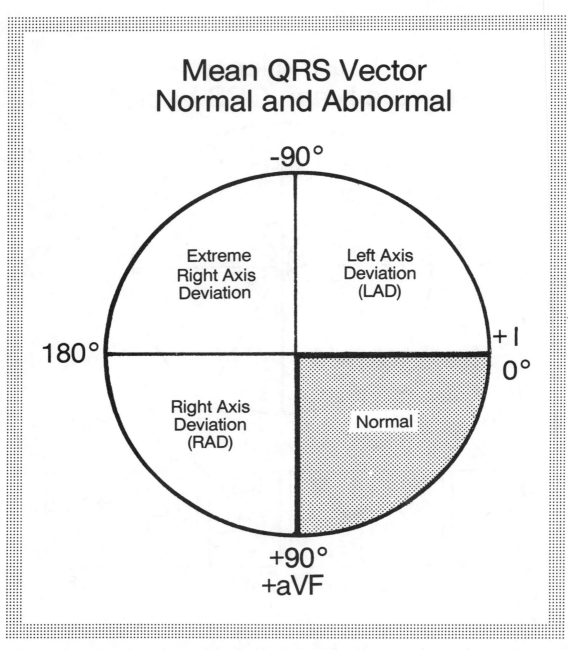

In the normal adult the mean QRS vector is usually between 0° and 90°, that is, the mean QRS vector is normally between leads I and aVF (shaded area). From 0° to −90° is *left axis deviation (LAD)* and from *90° to 180°* is *right axis deviation (RAD)*. The area from −90° to 180° has usually been described as *extreme right axis deviation.*

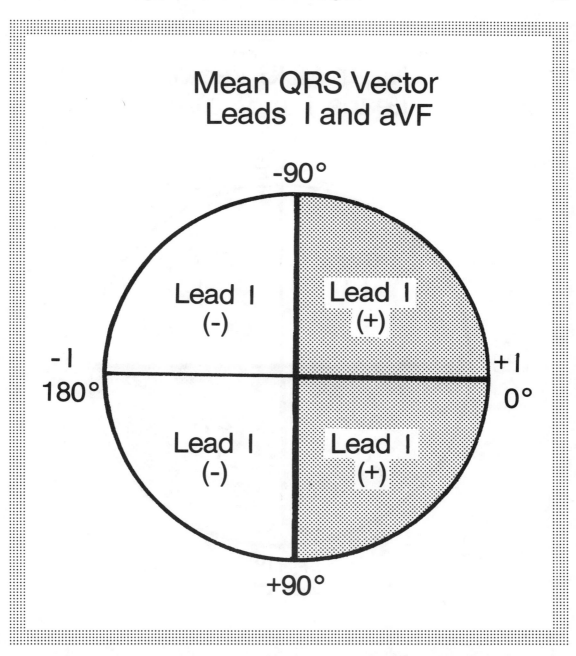

Since leads I and aVF are at right angles to each other, the quadrant in which a mean QRS vector is located may be easily found by using these two leads. The entire left (shaded) half of the circle is *positive* for lead I. Therefore, if the QRS complex is *positive* in lead I, the mean QRS vector is either normal or deviated to the left. If the QRS complex is *negative* in lead I, we have right axis or extreme right axis deviation.

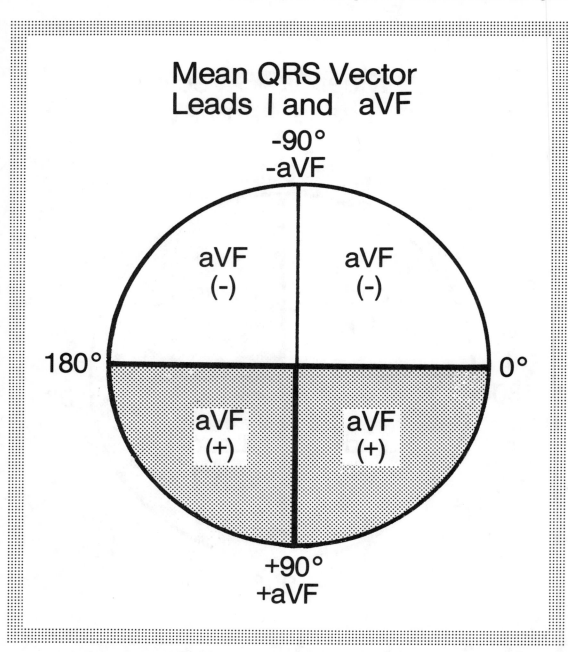

The entire lower half (shaded) of the circle is *positive* for lead aVF and the upper half is *negative* for lead aVF. Therefore, if the QRS complex is *positive* in lead aVF, the mean QRS vector is either normal or deviated to the right. If the QRS complex is *negative,* we have left axis deviation or extreme right axis deviation.

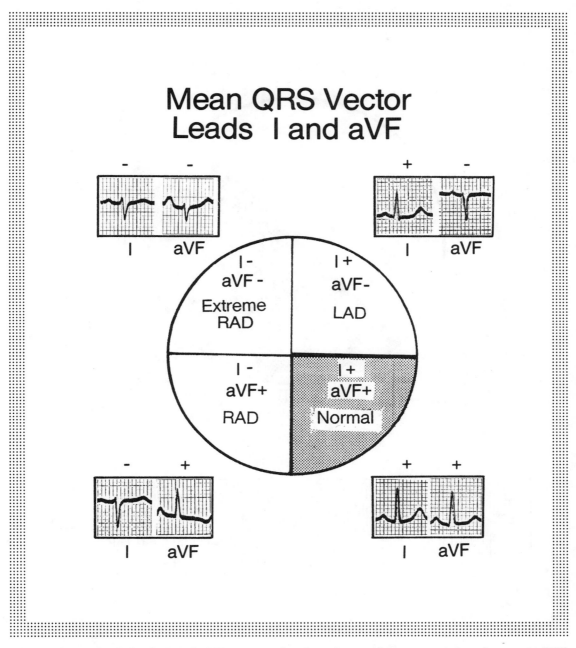

Mean QRS Vector Leads I and aVF

By utilizing both leads I and aVF, we can localize the quadrant containing the mean QRS vector. If both leads I and aVF are *positive*, the mean QRS vector is normal (shaded area). Describe leads I and aVF in left axis deviation, right axis deviation and extreme right axis deviation.

Mean T Vector

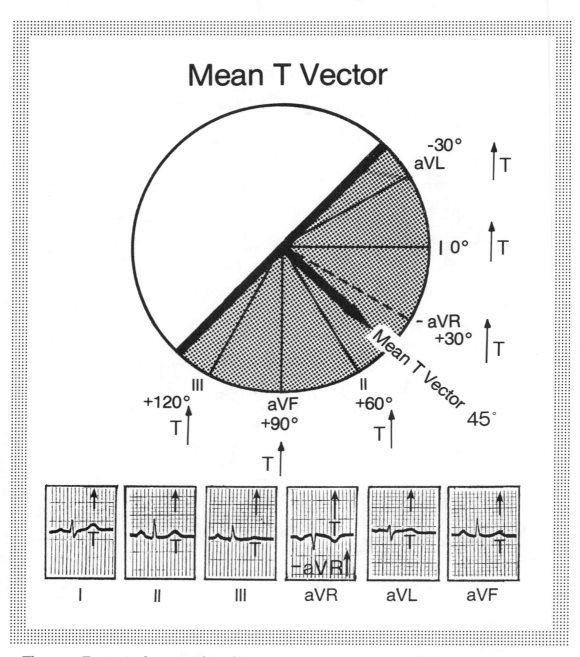

The *mean T vector* is determined in the same manner as the mean QRS vector. In the above illustration the T waves are positive in all the leads, including negative aVR (shaded area). The transition for the T wave bypasses all the leads. The mean T vector is perpendicular to the transition, on the positive side, at approximately 45° (large arrow).

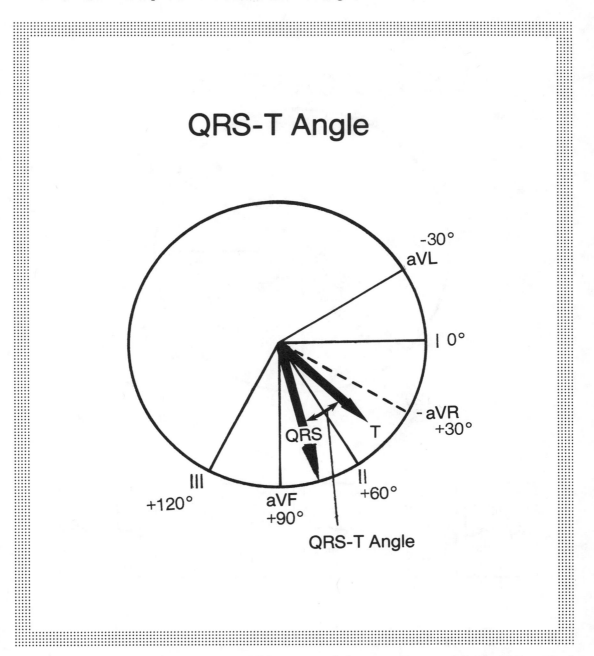

QRS-T Angle

The angle formed between the mean QRS vector and the mean T vector is a sensitive method for relating the forces of ventricular depolarization to the forces of ventricular repolarization. In the normal adult the *QRS-T angle* is rarely greater than 60° and often less than 45°. In the above illustration, using the same electrocardiogram as on the previous page, we find the QRS-T angle to be 30°.

Normal QRS-T Angle

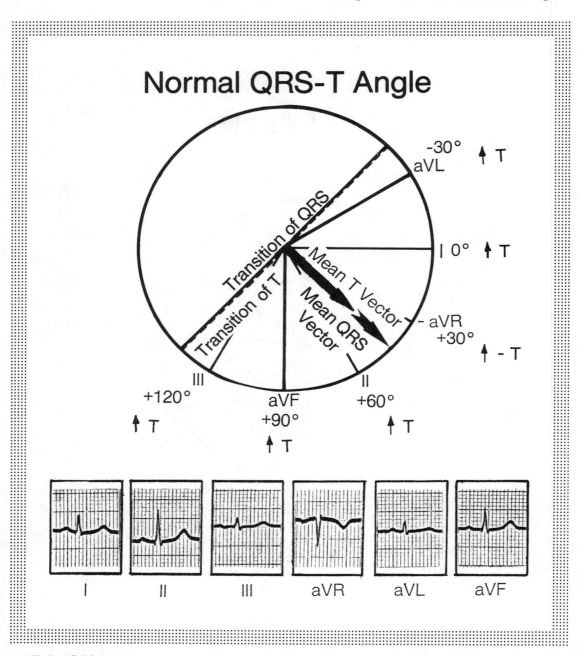

All the QRS complexes are positive, as are all the T waves. The mean QRS vector and the mean T vector are superimposed, thereby forming a very narrow, if any, angle between them. For the QRS-T angle to be normally narrow the T wave should have the *same* orientation as the QRS complex (e.g., both positive) in leads I, II and aVF. If not, stop and calculate. It may still be within normal limits. On the next two pages are examples of a wide and a very wide QRS-T angle.

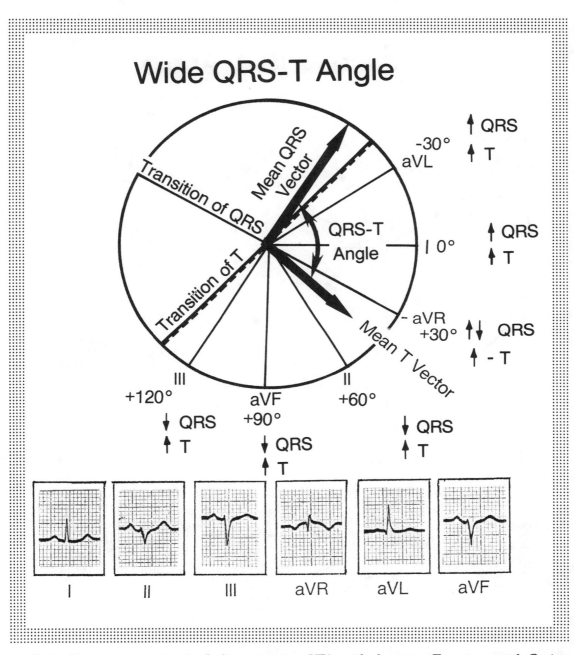

All the T waves are *positive* (including negative aVR), with the mean T vector at 45°. Owing to the marked left axis deviation of the mean QRS vector (−60°), a wide angle is formed between the mean QRS vector and the mean T vector (105°). Note: The T wave does not have the same orientation as the QRS complex in leads II and aVF.

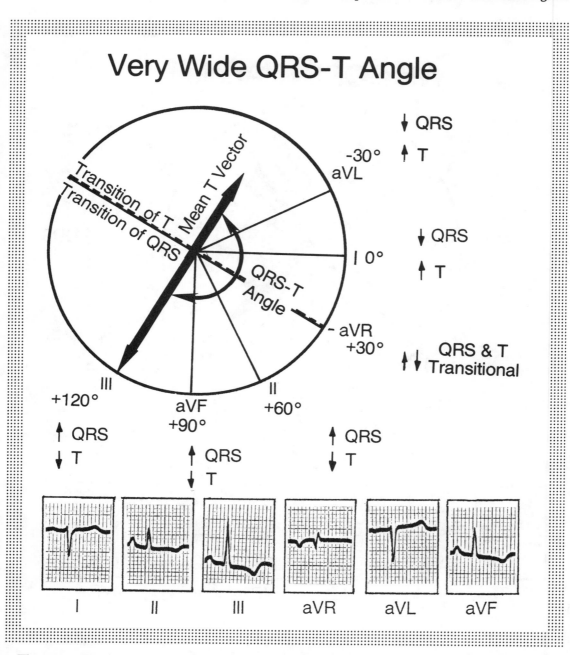

The transitional zone for both the mean QRS vector and the mean T vector is at lead aVR. In all other leads the QRS deflections are opposite the T wave deflections. The right axis deviation of the mean QRS vector (120°) and the left axis deviation (−60°) of the mean T vector result in a very wide QRS-T angle (180°).

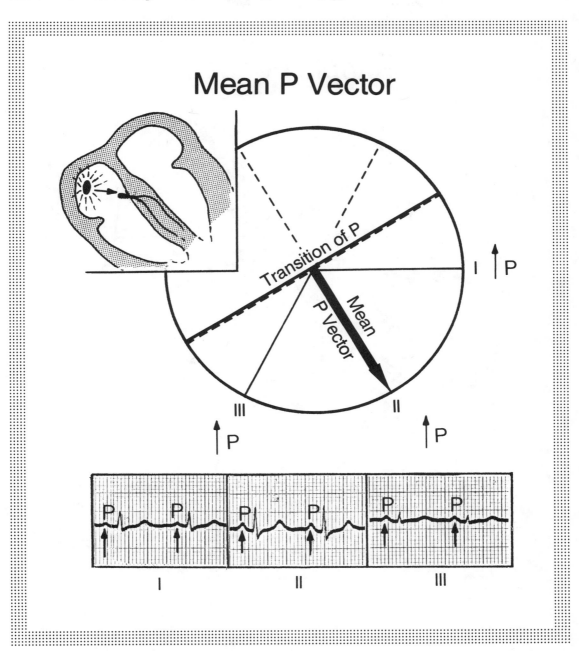

To find the *mean P vector,* use the same approach as for the mean QRS and T vectors. Note above that the mean P vector is along the axis of lead II at 60°. The normal range for the mean P vector is between 0° and 90°, similar to the normal range for the mean QRS vector. Therefore, the P waves in normal sinus rhythm are usually *positive* in leads I, II and aVF.

Ectopic Focus

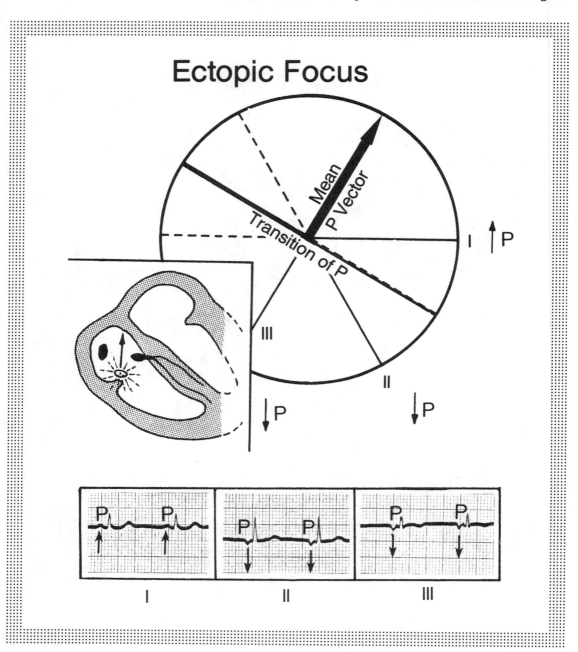

The P wave is *positive* in lead I but *negative* in leads II and III. The transition is, therefore, between leads I and II, with an abnormal deviation of the mean P vector. Thus the electrical impulse is not from the SA node but from some other focus; it is from an *ectopic focus* representing an abnormal sequence of atrial depolarization.

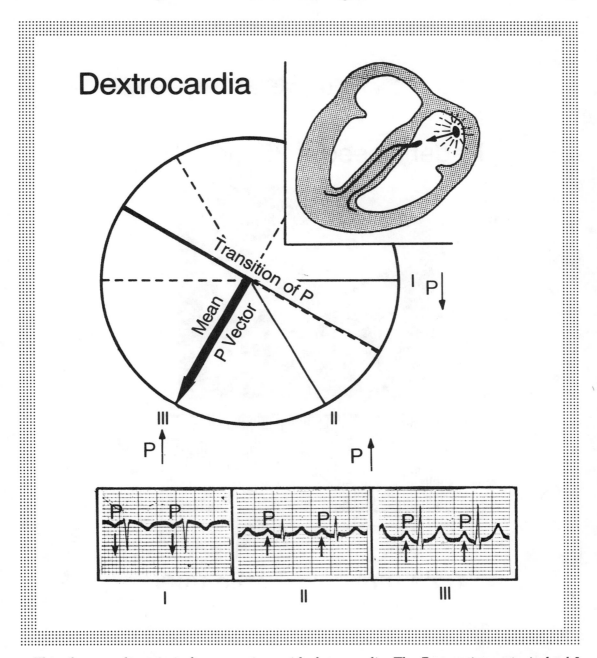

Dextrocardia

This electrocardiogram is from a patient with dextrocardia. The P wave is *negative* in lead I but *positive* in leads II and III. The mean P vector is deviated abnormally to the right. Another more common cause of a negative P wave in lead I is the reversal of electrodes in lead I (positive on the right arm and negative on the left).

Heart Rate

Paper Speed = 25 mm./sec.

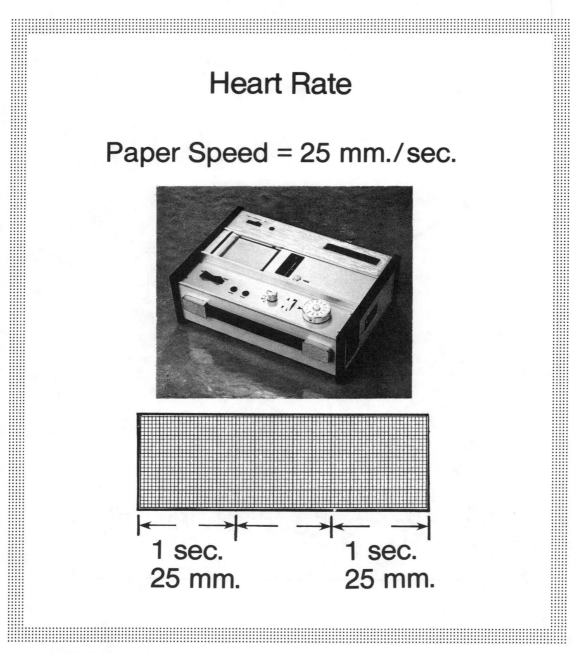

The determination of heart rate from the electrocardiogram depends on the speed of the paper when recording the electrocardiogram. The usual speed of the paper is *25 mm (five large boxes) per second.* Whenever the paper speed is changed, which is possible on most machines, it should be indicated on the electrocardiogram.

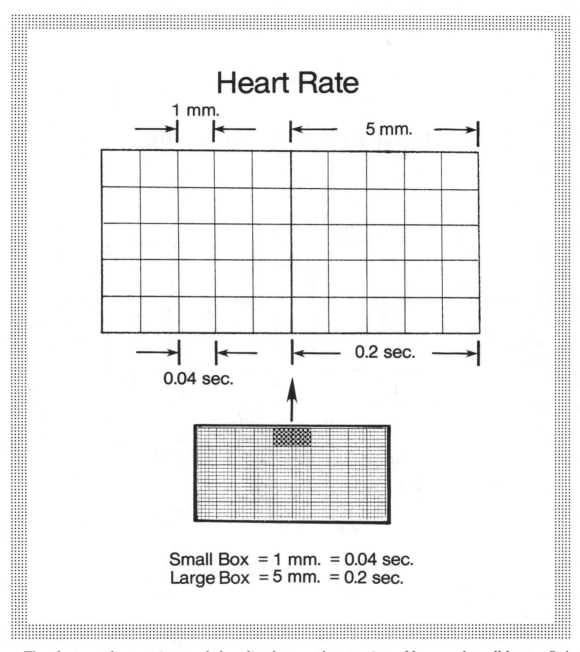

Heart Rate

Small Box = 1 mm. = 0.04 sec.
Large Box = 5 mm. = 0.2 sec.

The electrocardiogram is recorded on lined paper that consists of large and small boxes. *Each large box measures 5mm.* and *each small box 1 mm.* At the paper speed of 25 mm. per second, *each large box represents 0.2 second* and *each small box 0.04 second.*

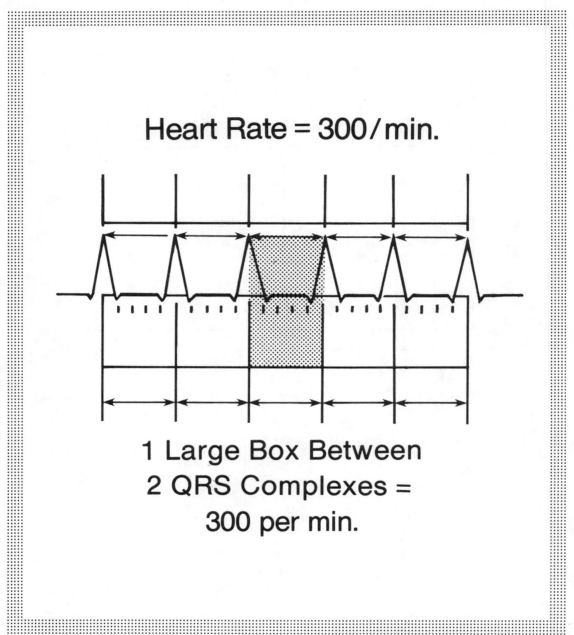

At the usual paper speed of 25 mm. per second (five large boxes), when the heart rate is *300 per minute* the interval is *one large box (5mm., 0.2 second) between two QRS complexes.* All that is necessary to determine heart rate when the rhythm is regular is to count the number of large boxes between two QRS complexes and divide into 300.

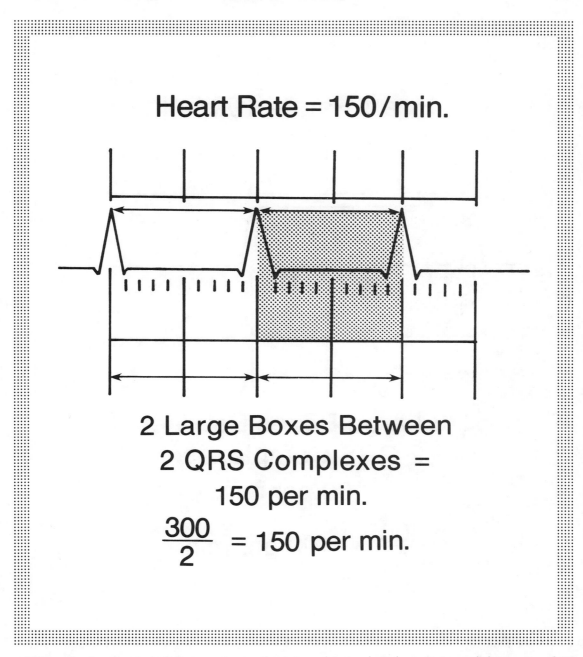

When the heart rate is 150 per minute, the interval is *two large boxes (0.4 second) between two QRS complexes (300/2).* This determination is facilitated if you start the count with a QRS complex or P wave, whichever you are measuring, that falls on a heavy line.

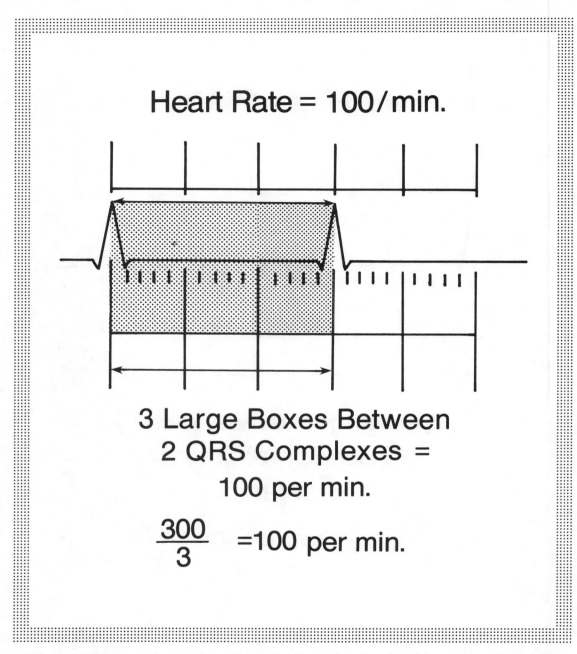

Heart Rate = 100/min.

3 Large Boxes Between
2 QRS Complexes =
100 per min.

$$\frac{300}{3} = 100 \text{ per min.}$$

When the heart rate is 100 per minute, the interval is *three large boxes (0.6 second) between two QRS complexes (300/3)*. This method permits a rapid determination of heart rate when the rhythm is regular.

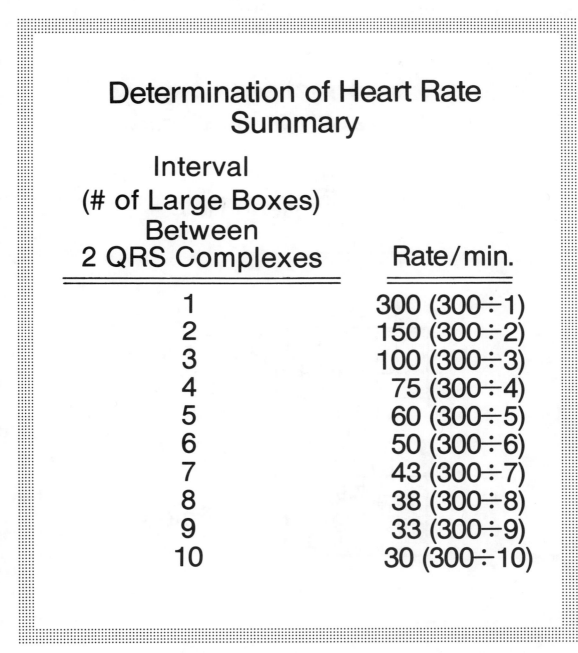

Determination of Heart Rate Summary

Interval (# of Large Boxes) Between 2 QRS Complexes	Rate/min.
1	300 (300÷1)
2	150 (300÷2)
3	100 (300÷3)
4	75 (300÷4)
5	60 (300÷5)
6	50 (300÷6)
7	43 (300÷7)
8	38 (300÷8)
9	33 (300÷9)
10	30 (300÷10)

This relationship permits the determination of heart rate using only two QRS complexes when the rhythm is regular. Simply count the number of large boxes and any fraction, and divide into 300 for the heart rate. When the rhythm is irregular, you have to count numerous QRS complexes to arrive at the proper average.

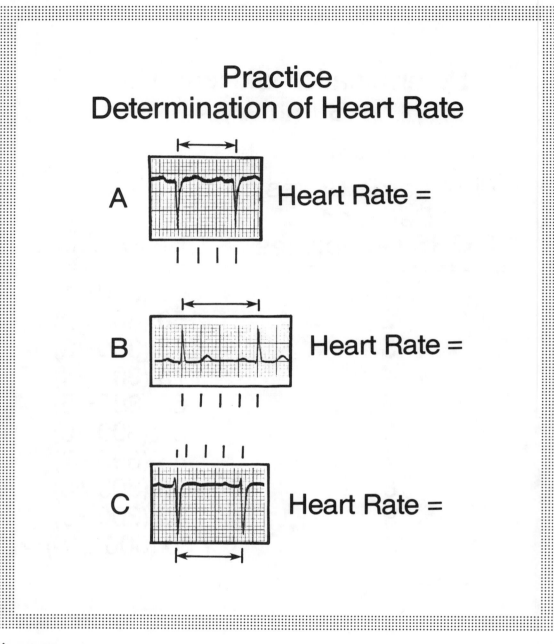

Practice
Determination of Heart Rate

A   Heart Rate =

B   Heart Rate =

C   Heart Rate =

Answers:

A. Three large boxes between two QRS complexes: heart rate = 100 per minute($300 \div 3 = 100$).

B. Four large boxes between two QRS complexes: heart rate = 75 per minute($300 \div 4 = 75$).

C. Three and a half large boxes between two QRS complexes: heart rate = 86 per minute ($300 \div 3.5 = 86$).

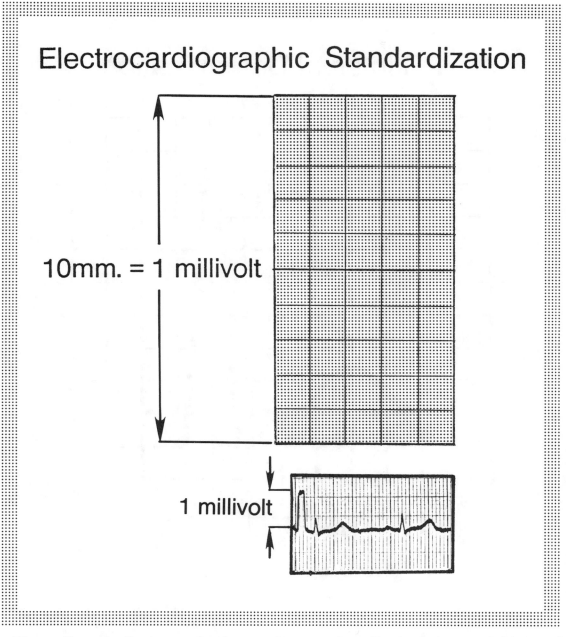

The usual standardization on the electrocardiogram of 1 millivolt results in a deflection of two large boxes (10 mm.) The standardization is essential in order to properly evaluate the size of the deflections.

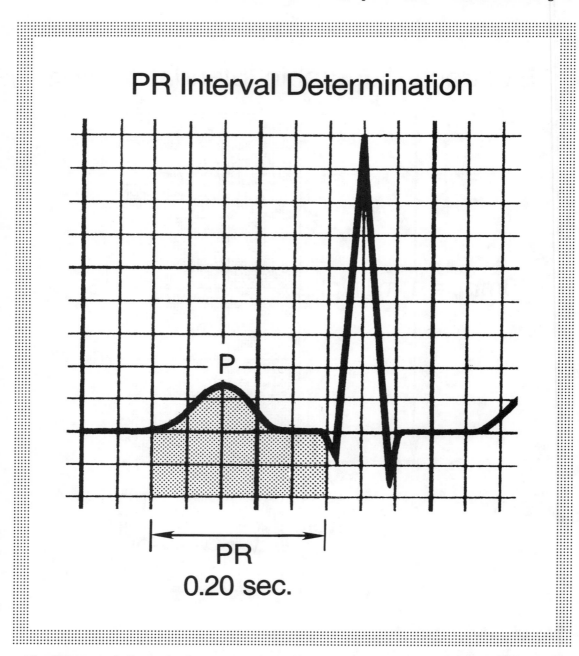

The PR interval (from the beginning of the P wave to the beginning of the QRS complex) is 0.20 second (five small boxes or one large box). *The normal PR interval is from 0.12 to 0.20 second.* This is an important measurement, since an abnormal prolongation represents a problem in the transmission of the electrical impulse from the atria to the ventricles.

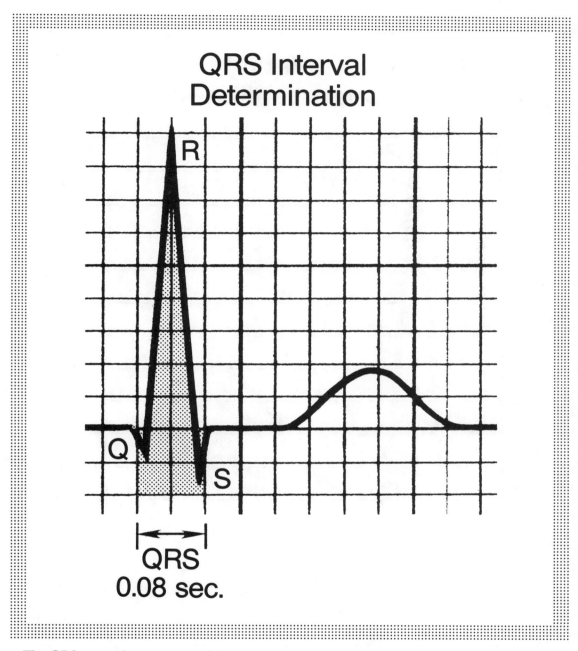

The QRS interval is 0.08 second (two small boxes). *The normal interval for ventricular depolarization is 0.08 second.* Abnormal prolongation represents an intraventricular conduction disturbance. QRS interval prolongation is seen in right and left bundle branch block. These will be studied in a later chapter.

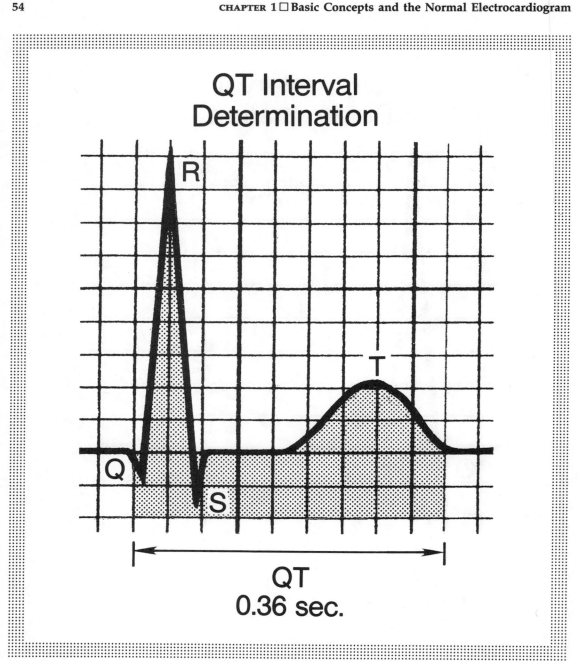

The *QT interval,* representing the depolarization and repolarization of the ventricles, is rate-dependent.

Heart Rate (beats per minute)	QT Interval (sec.)
40	0.46
60	0.39
80	0.35
100	0.31
120	0.29
140	0.26
160	0.25

Various metabolic abnormalities may alter the QT interval.

Normal Sinus Rhythm

1. Normal Mean P Vector (to the left and inferior - upright P waves in leads I and aVF or I and II.

2. Each P wave must be followed by a QRS complex and each QRS complex must be preceded by a P wave.

3. The normal PR interval (from the beginning of the P wave to the beginning of the QRS complex) is rarely greater than 0.2 sec. (one large box) in duration. The normal range is 0.12 to 0.2 sec. and is constant from beat to beat.

4. The rate is constant between 60 and 100 beats per minute.

In order to describe the rhythm of the heart as *sinus rhythm* (the impulse originating in the sinoatrial node, which is the normal pacemaker of the heart) without qualifications, the above requirements must be met.

The Frontal Plane

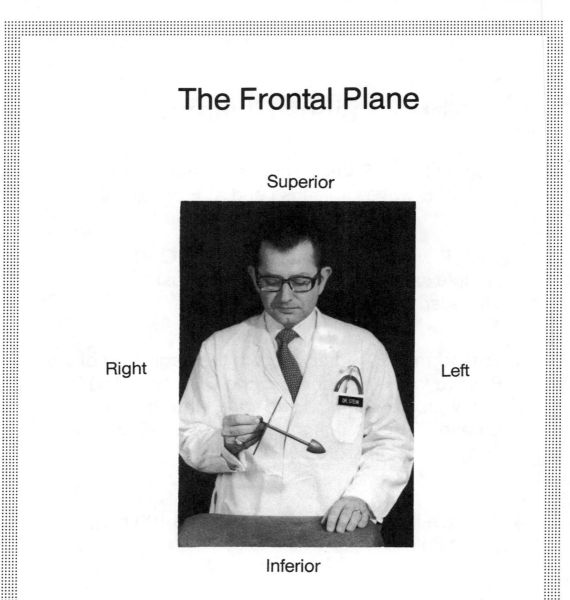

The six electrocardiographic leads studied heretofore—I, II, III, aVR, aVL and aVF—are leads in the *frontal plane.* The boundaries of the frontal plane are *superior, inferior, right and left.*

We are still missing the third dimension, since the cardiac vector is three-dimensional.

Frontal Plane Vectors

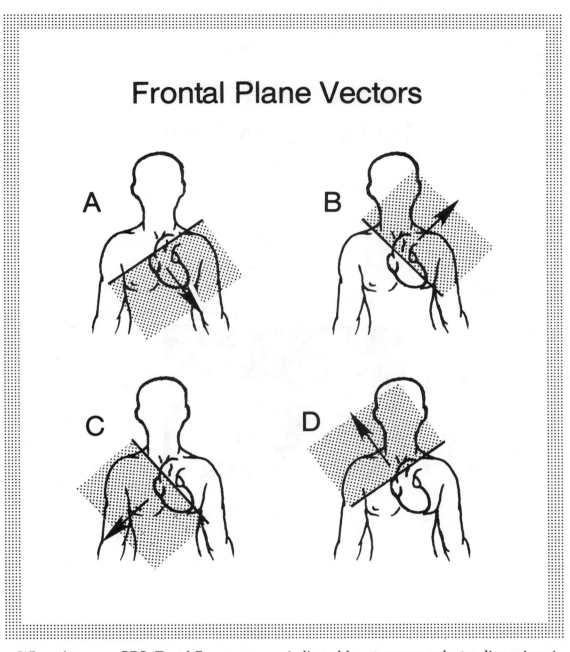

When the mean QRS, T and P vectors were indicated by an arrow, only *two* dimensions in space could be described.

A. The arrow points to the *left* and *inferiorly.*

B. The arrow points to the *left* and *superiorly.*

C. The arrow points to the *right* and *inferiorly.*

D. The arrow points to the *right* and *superiorly.*

The Horizontal Plane

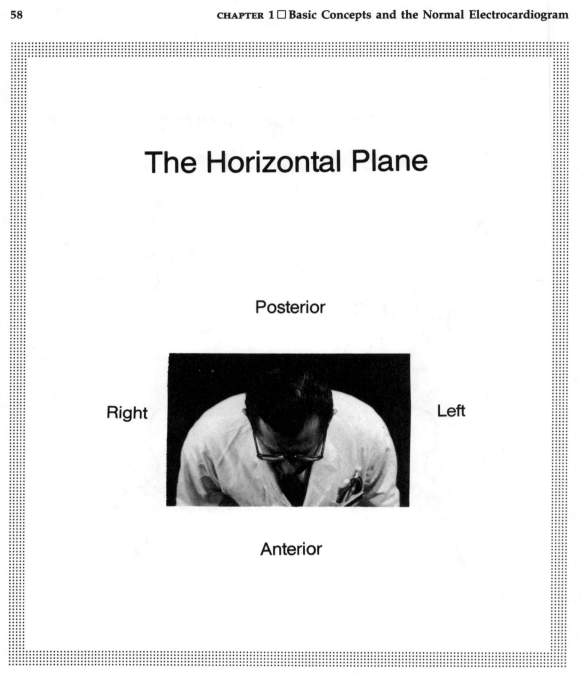

In order to provide the third dimension in space to describe the cardiac vectors, the *horizontal* plane must be added. The boundaries of the horizontal plane are *anterior, posterior, right and left*. After many years and many trials, the chest or precordial leads were established. Still later, measurements of the cardiac vectors in the horizontal plane were shown to be possible. Precordial electrodes were placed across the chest.

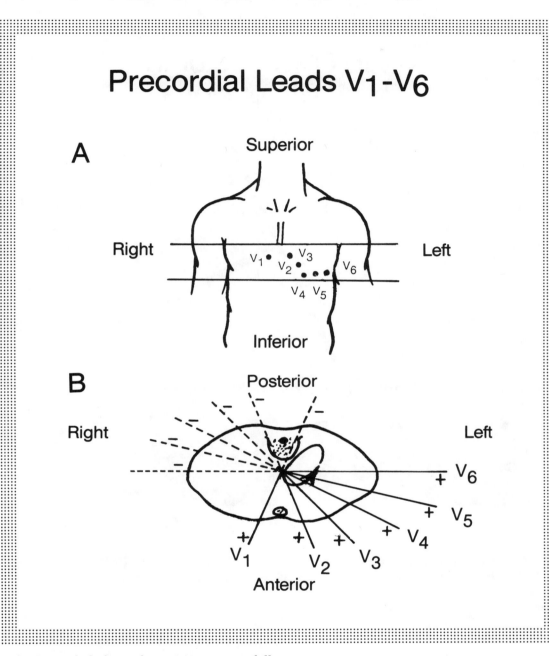

Precordial Leads V₁-V₆

A. Precordial electrode positions are as follows:
  V_1 Fourth intercostal space to the right of the sternum.
  V_2 Fourth intercostal space to the left of the sternum.
  V_3 Midway between V_2 and V_4.
  V_4 Fifth intercostal space—midclavicular line.
  V_5 Anterior axillary line—horizontal level of V_4.
  V_6 Midaxillary line—horizontal level of V_4.
B. QRS loop in the horizontal plane.

Mean QRS Vector in Three Dimensions

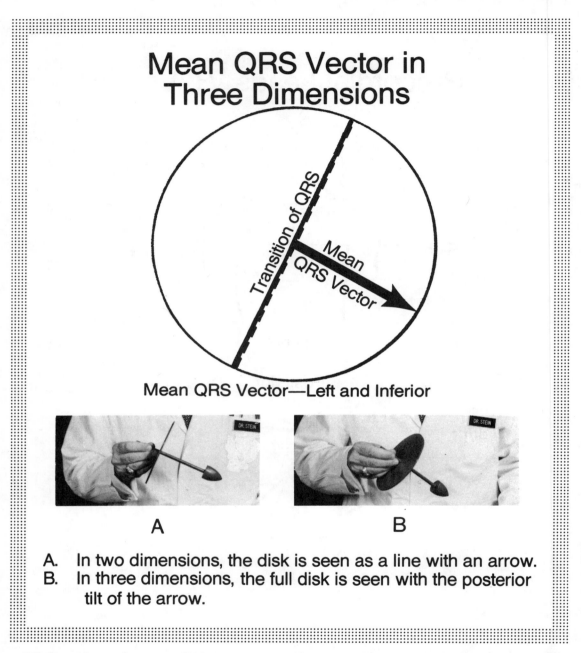

Transition of QRS

Mean QRS Vector

Mean QRS Vector—Left and Inferior

A   B

A.   In two dimensions, the disk is seen as a line with an arrow.
B.   In three dimensions, the full disk is seen with the posterior tilt of the arrow.

While studying the mean QRS vector in the frontal plane, we were accustomed to seeing a line and an arrow. We had not really been looking at a transitional *line* but at a *disk* dividing the body into positive and negative areas. The circumference of this disk, viewed on end, appeared to be a line (A). In a three-dimensional view, as seen in B, the disk and arrow are tilted slightly posteriorly to show that we are not actually looking at a line, but at a disk.

Vectorial Concept in Three Dimensions

Vector Model

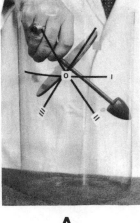

A

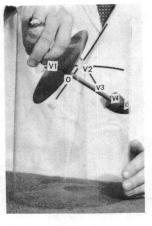

B

A. Frontal leads   B. Horizontal leads

The vector model may be used to better visualize the cardiac vector in three dimensions. The lines in A, representing the *frontal* plane, are leads I, II and III. The precordial leads in B, representing the *horizontal* plane, are leads V_1 to V_6. The zero on the frontal plane and the zero on the horizontal plane line up, and they line up with the center point of the disk. *We can rotate the disk only through the zero point,* which limits its motion. This method facilitates the understanding of the general vectorial concept in three dimensions.

Stepwise Determination of Mean QRS Vector in Three Dimensions

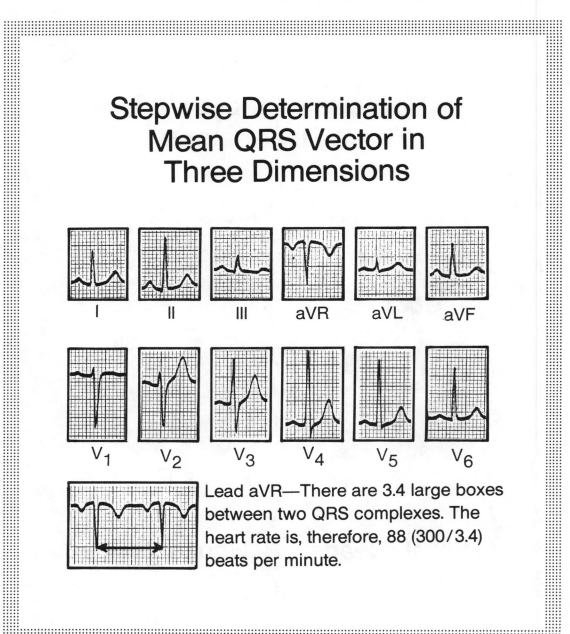

Lead aVR—There are 3.4 large boxes between two QRS complexes. The heart rate is, therefore, 88 (300/3.4) beats per minute.

This electrocardiogram is analyzed on the next three pages as to the mean QRS vector in three dimensions. We will first determine the mean QRS vector in the frontal plane, using leads I, II, III, aVR, aVL and aVF. Then we will examine the contribution of the precordial (chest) leads, V_1 to V_6, to our understanding of the mean QRS vector in three dimensions.

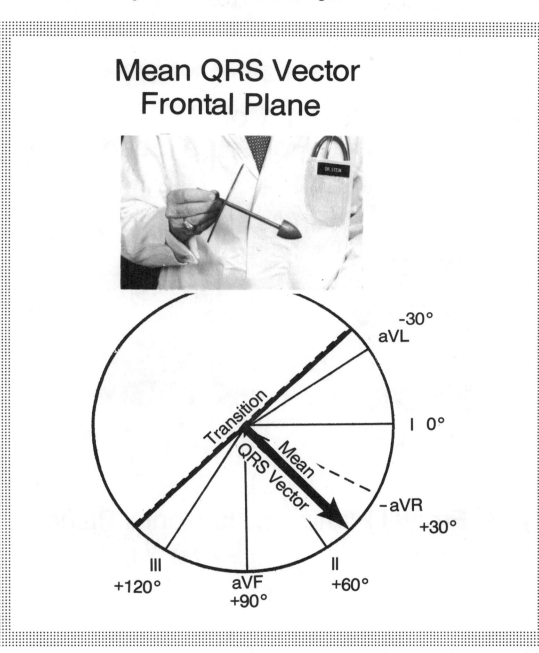

Mean QRS Vector
Frontal Plane

All six leads are positive, remembering to invert lead aVR. The transitional zone bypasses all of the leads, and the mean QRS vector falls between leads II and aVR, to the *left* and *inferiorly* in the frontal plane. The disk and arrow, held to the left and inferiorly, do not actually appear as a disk and an arrow but rather as a line and an arrow.

Vector Model
Frontal and Horizontal Leads

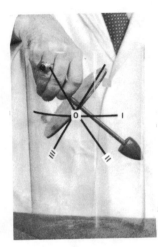 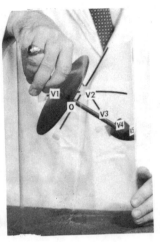

A   B

A. Frontal Plane   B. Horizontal Plane
Leads I, II, III   Leads V_1-V_6

Using our vector model in A we see leads I, II and III, and the vector is to the *left* and *inferior*. In B, on the other side of the model, we have a representation of the horizontal plane. *If there were no anterior-posterior rotation,* if the vector were simply to the *left* and *inferior,* lead V_1 would be *negative.* (V_1 is the only precordial lead on the negative side of the disk. The arrow side of the disk is the positive side.) Leads V_2, V_3, V_4, V_5 and V_6 would all be positive. Is this the case in the electrocardiogram on page 62? NO....

Mean QRS Vector in Three Dimensions

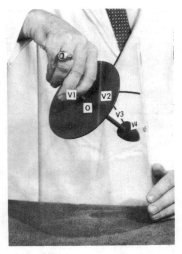

Left, Inferior, and Posterior

On looking again at page 62, we see that not only lead V_1 but also V_2 is *negative*. Leads V_3, V_4, V_5 and V_6 are *positive*. The transition in the horizontal plane is between leads V_2 and V_3. How do we make our model reflect the electrocardiographic inscription? We must tilt the disk so that the arrow faces *posteriorly*. In this position both leads V_1 and V_2 are negative. Leads V_3 through V_6 are positive.

The mean QRS vector, in three dimensions, is to the *left, inferior* and *posterior*. This describes the normal adult mean QRS vector.

Stepwise Determination of Mean QRS Vector in Three Dimensions

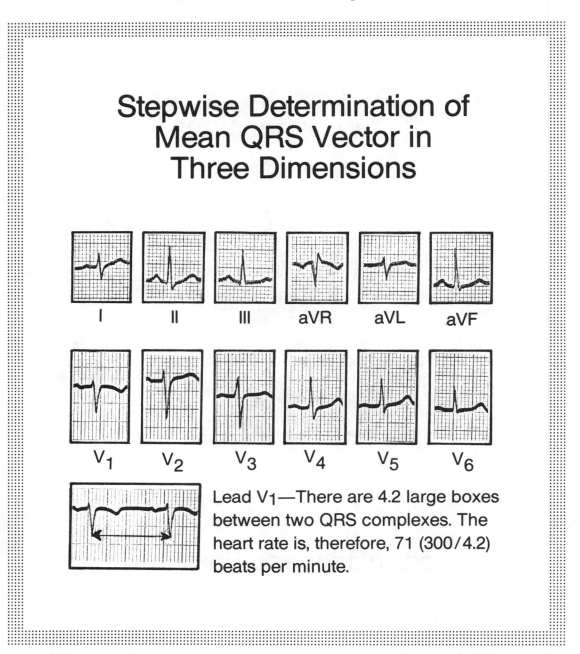

Lead V₁—There are 4.2 large boxes between two QRS complexes. The heart rate is, therefore, 71 (300/4.2) beats per minute.

As we did with the previous electrocardiogram, we will analyze the mean QRS vector in three dimensions on the next three pages.

To summarize, whether the mean QRS vector is *left and inferior, left and superior, right and inferior* or *right and superior* is determined by the *frontal plane leads*, I, II, III, aVR, aVL and aVF. Whether the mean QRS vector is *anterior* or *posterior* must be determined from the *horizontal plane leads*, V₁ to V₆.

Mean QRS Vector at 90⁰

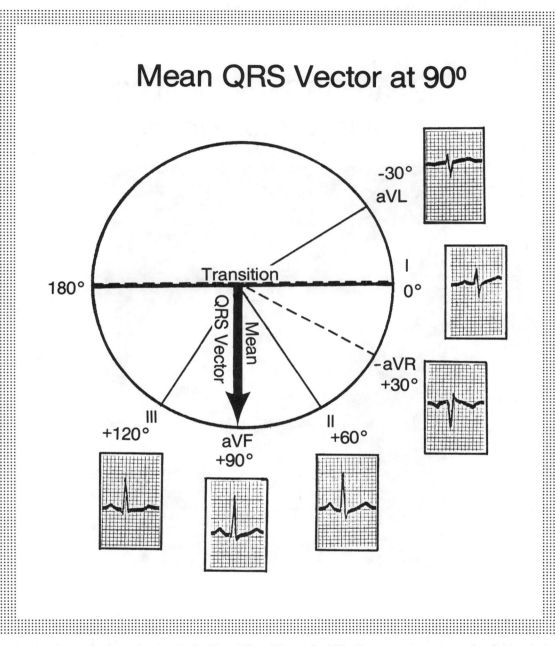

In the frontal plane leads, I, II, III, aVR, aVL and aVF, the transition is at lead I and the mean QRS vector is at 90°. The mean QRS vector in the frontal plane is neither to the left nor to the right. The arrow is pointing inferiorly.

Mean QRS Vector at 90⁰
Using Vector Model

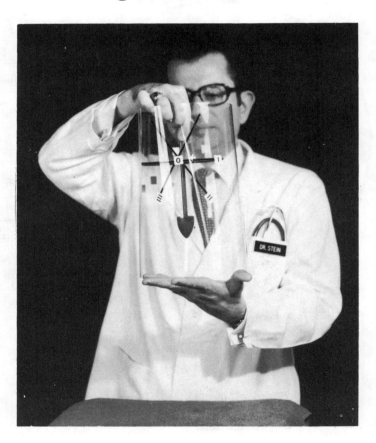

The vector model is very useful in enabling us to visualize the mean QRS vector in three dimensions. Here we are looking at the frontal plane leads, I, II and III. The transition is at lead I, 0°, and the mean QRS vector is perpendicular to it at lead aVF, 90°.

Vector Model-Horizontal Plane

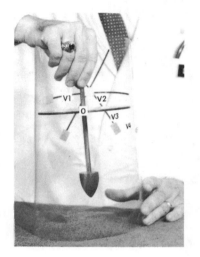

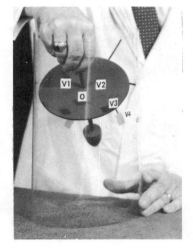

A   B

Horizontal Plane Leads V$_1$-V$_6$

A. If the mean QRS vector were directly inferior, neither anterior nor posterior, then leads V$_1$ and V$_2$ would both be negative and leads V$_3$ to V$_6$ would be positive.

B. The electrocardiogram on page 66, however, shows the transition to be between leads V$_3$ and V$_4$. In order to make lead V$_3$ negative on the vector model, we must tilt the arrow posteriorly. The mean QRS vector is, therefore, inferior and posterior in three dimensions.

Normal Mean QRS Vector in Three Dimensions

A

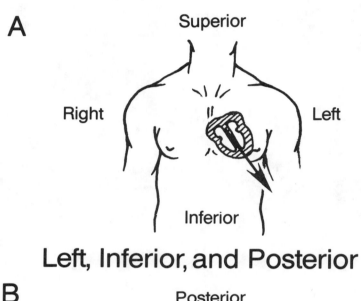

Left, Inferior, and Posterior

B

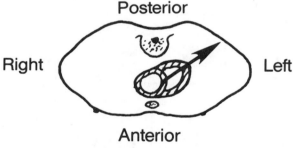

To summarize, the *normal* mean QRS vector in the *frontal* plane (A) is oriented to the *left* and *inferiorly*. In the *horizontal* plane (B), we see that it is also *posterior*.

The vector approach affords us a unifying concept in our understanding of the electrocardiogram. By visualizing the distribution of electrical potential in a three-dimensional way, a single picture actually indicates what we will find on the 12 lead electrocardiogram.

Abnormal Electrocardiogram Stepwise Determination of Mean QRS Vector in Three Dimensions

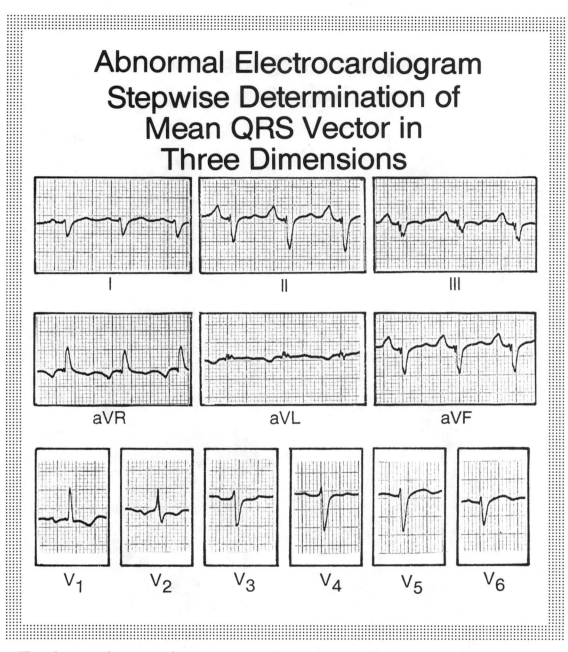

This electrocardiogram is from a patient with chronic lung disease and resulting heart failure (cor pulmonale), with hypertrophy of the right atrium and right ventricle. These entities will be studied in the next chapter. For the present, we will evaluate the mean QRS vector, as we have done in previous electrocardiograms.

Mean QRS Vector
Right, Superior, Anterior

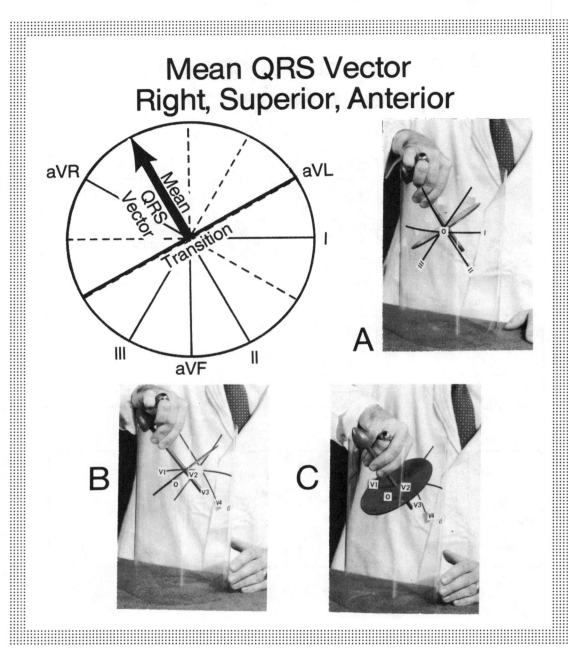

A. In the frontal plane the mean QRS vector is to the *right* and *superior,* with leads I, II and III negative, facing away from the arrow side of the disk.

B. If the mean QRS vector were merely to the right and superior, lead V_1 would be positive and V_2 to V_6 would fall on the negative side of the disk.

C. The electrocardiogram (p. 71), however, reveals that the transition is between leads V_2 and V_3. We must tilt the disk so that the arrow points *anteriorly.* The mean QRS vector, therefore, is to the *right, superior* and *anterior.*

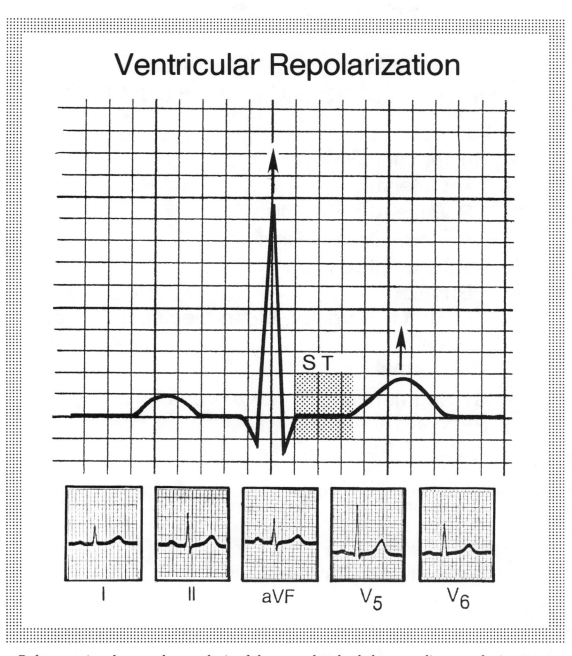

Ventricular Repolarization

S T

I   II   aVF   V₅   V₆

Before starting the complete analysis of the normal 12 lead electrocardiogram, the importance of the phase of ventricular repolarization must again be emphasized.

1. The ST segment is normally isoelectric, neither elevated nor depressed, at the same level as the resting baseline. The ST segment may, however, slope upward toward a tall T wave.

2. In order to have a normal QRS-T angle in *three dimensions*, the T wave is in the same direction (upward, positive, arrows above) as the QRS complex in leads I, II, aVF, V₅ and V₆.

Electrocardiographic Interpretation

1. Rhythm and Rate
       PR Interval
       P Wave Abnormalities
       Abnormalities of Rhythm
2. QRS Complex
       Duration
       Mean QRS Vector, Mean Electrical Axis or
       "Axis"
       Abnormalities
3. ST Segment and T Wave (Ventricular
    Repolarization)
       QRS-T Angle
       Abnormalities
4. QT Interval

Impression and Comment

Utilizing all the information studied so far, we can analyze electrocardiograms according to the four steps enumerated above.

Practice
ECG Analysis

Practice
ECG Analysis

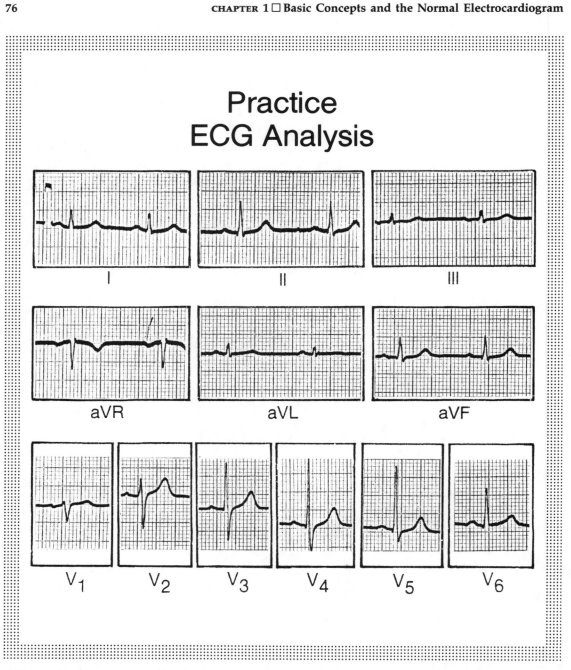

Using the four steps outlined on page 74, analyze this and the next electrocardiogram. After you have completed each analysis, compare with the review on the following page.

The patient is a healthy adult.

Analysis:

ECG ANALYSIS

1. Rhythm and Rate
   Rhythm: Sinus Rhythm
   Rate: 65/min.
   PR Interval: 0.16 sec.
2. QRS Complex
   Duration: 0.08 sec.
   Axis: +45°
3. Ventricular Repolarization
   ST Segment: Neither significantly elevated nor depressed
   T Wave: QRS-T angle normal
4. QT Interval: 0.38 sec.

Impression and Comment

Normal Electrocardiogram

Practice
ECG Analysis

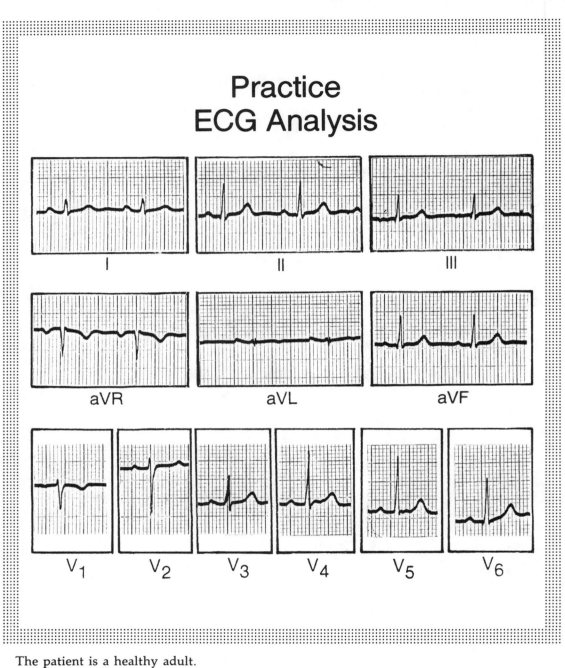

The patient is a healthy adult.

Analysis:

ECG ANALYSIS

1. Rhythm and Rate
   Rhythm: Sinus Rhythm
   Rate: 75/min.
   PR Interval: 0.18 sec.
2. QRS Complex
   Duration: 0.08 sec.
   Axis: $+60°$
3. Ventricular Repolarization
   ST Segment: Neither significantly elevated nor depressed
   T Wave: QRS-T angle normal
4. QT Interval: 0.36 sec.

Impression and Comment

Normal Electrocardiogram

Chapter 2

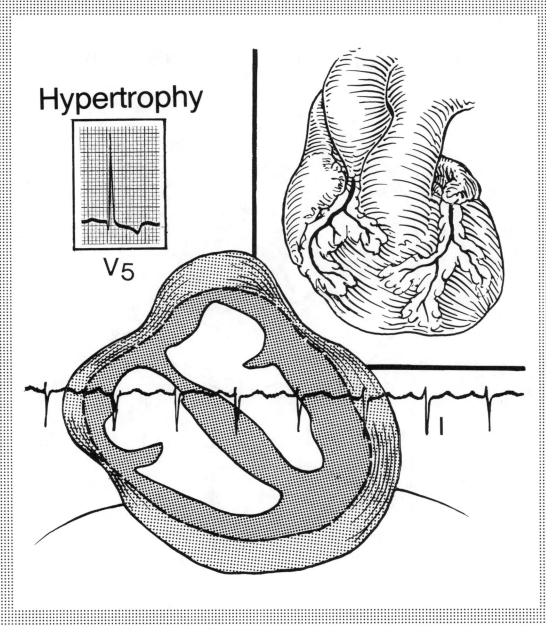

Hypertrophy

V_5

Myocardial hypertrophy refers to an increase in the muscular wall thickness of a chamber of the heart. The word *hypertrophy* is commonly used. However, hypertrophy is not the only cause of an enlarged chamber, and differentiation is often difficult on the electrocardiogram. *Enlargement* is a more inclusive term.

Right Ventricular Hypertrophy

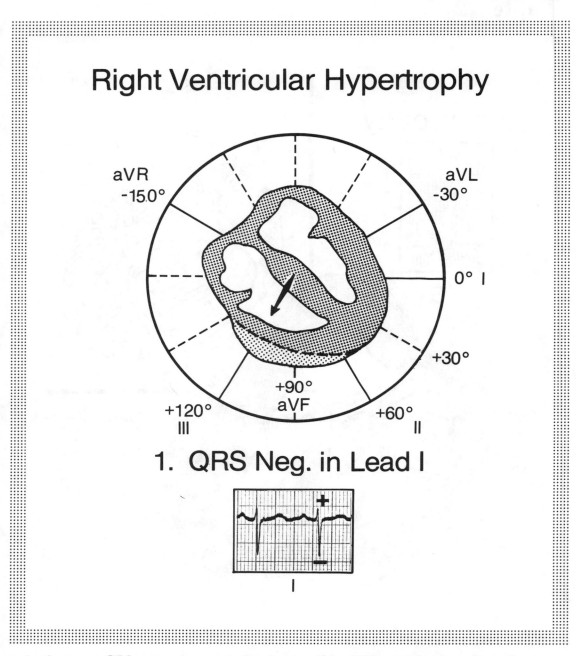

1. QRS Neg. in Lead I

As the mean QRS vector (mean electrical axis of the QRS) shifts rightward, it faces *away* from lead I, inscribing a QRS complex in lead I that is *predominantly negative.* A predominantly negative QRS complex in lead I signifies right axis deviation. *Right axis deviation is a major electrocardiographic criterion of right ventricular hypertrophy.*

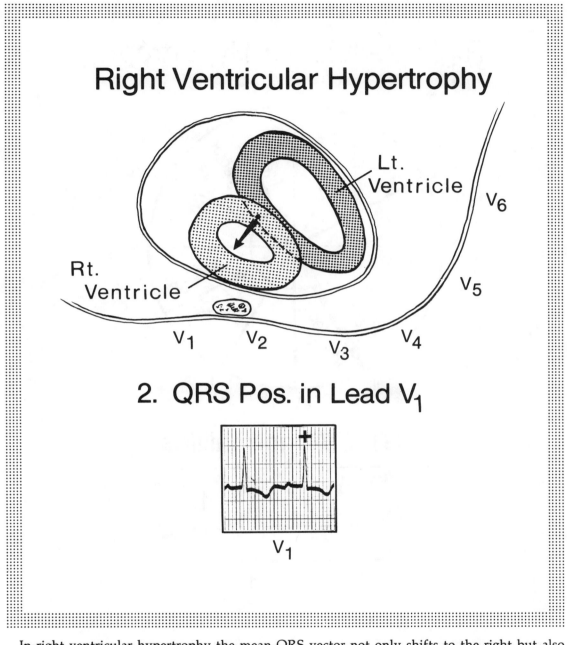

Right Ventricular Hypertrophy

Lt.
Ventricle

V_6

V_5

Rt.
Ventricle

V_1 V_2 V_3 V_4

2. QRS Pos. in Lead V_1

+

V_1

In right ventricular hypertrophy the mean QRS vector not only shifts to the right but also *anteriorly*. It therefore faces lead V_1, inscribing a predominantly *positive QRS complex in lead V_1. A predominantly positive QRS complex in lead V_1 is another major electrocardiographic criterion of right ventricular hypertrophy.*

Right Ventricular Hypertrophy

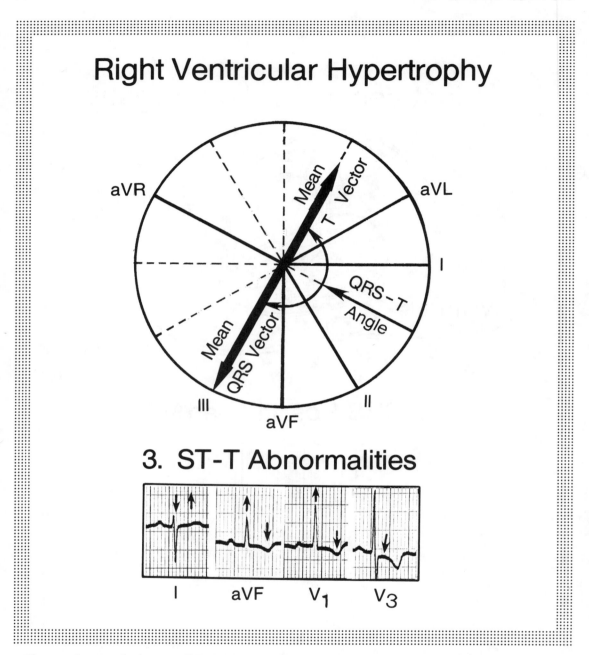

3. ST-T Abnormalities

Ventricular repolarization (ST-T) abnormalities are frequently seen in right ventricular hypertrophy. In the above electrocardiogram the QRS complexes and T waves are opposite in orientation. Where the QRS complex is positive the T wave is negative, and where the QRS is negative the T wave is positive. *The QRS-T angle is, therefore, very wide—180°.* ST segment depression is seen in lead V_3.

Right Ventricular Hypertrophy
Principal Criteria
Review

1. Neg. QRS in Lead I

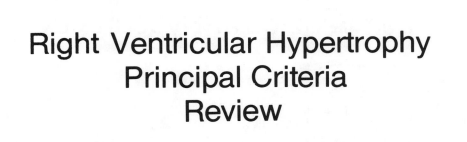

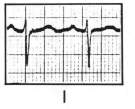

2. Pos. QRS in Lead V₁

I

V₁

3. ST-T Abnormalities

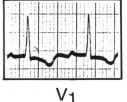

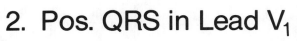

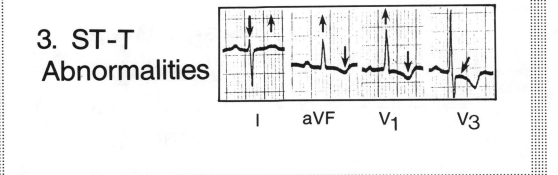

I   aVF   V₁   V₃

In right ventricular hypertrophy the mean QRS vector shifts *rightward* and *anteriorly*, inscribing both the *negative* QRS complex in lead I and the *positive* QRS complex in lead V_1. Ventricular repolarization (ST-T) abnormalities commonly accompany right ventricular hypertrophy.

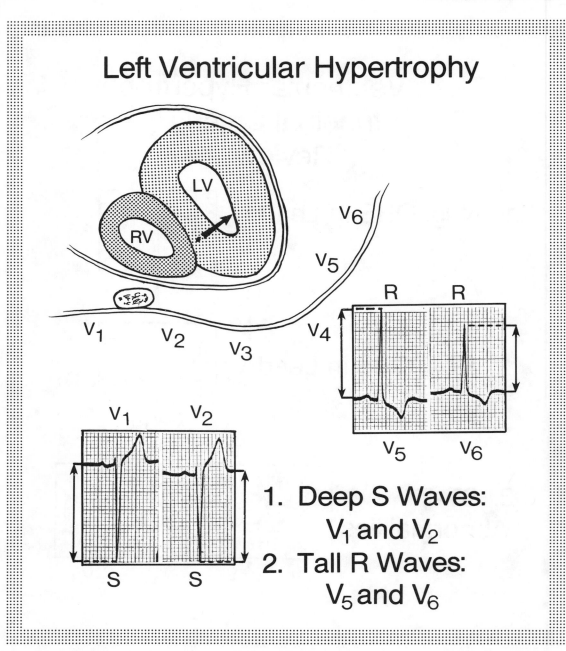

Left Ventricular Hypertrophy

1. Deep S Waves:
   V_1 and V_2
2. Tall R Waves:
   V_5 and V_6

In left ventricular hypertrophy the mean QRS vector, which is normally oriented to the left, inferiorly and posteriorly, is markedly accentuated, inscribing *deep S waves* in the right precordial leads (V_1 and V_2) and *tall R waves* in the left precordial leads (V_5 and V_6).

Left Ventricular Hypertrophy

1. Magnitude Criteria

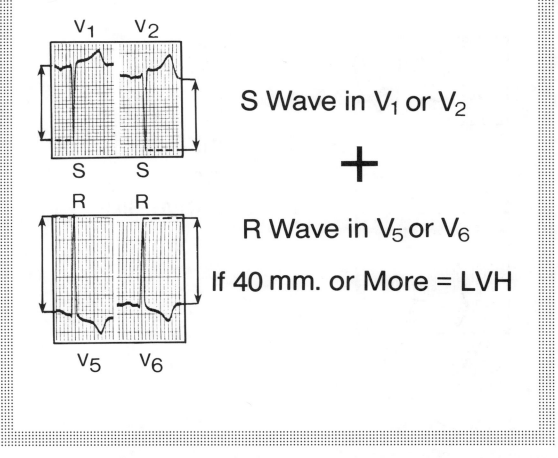

S Wave in V_1 or V_2

+

R Wave in V_5 or V_6

If 40 mm. or More = LVH

Increased magnitude of the QRS complex is the major electrocardiographic criterion of left ventricular hypertrophy in the adult. Because of the posterior orientation of the mean QRS vector in left ventricular hypertrophy, the increased magnitude is seen best in the precordial leads, V_1 to V_6. The diagnosis of left ventricular hypertrophy should not be made without evidence of increased magnitude. In addition, if any of the above leads (V_1, V_2, V_5, V_6) is greater than *30 mm.* alone (not in combination), left ventricular hypertrophy should be considered.

Left Ventricular Hypertrophy

2. ST-T Abnormalities

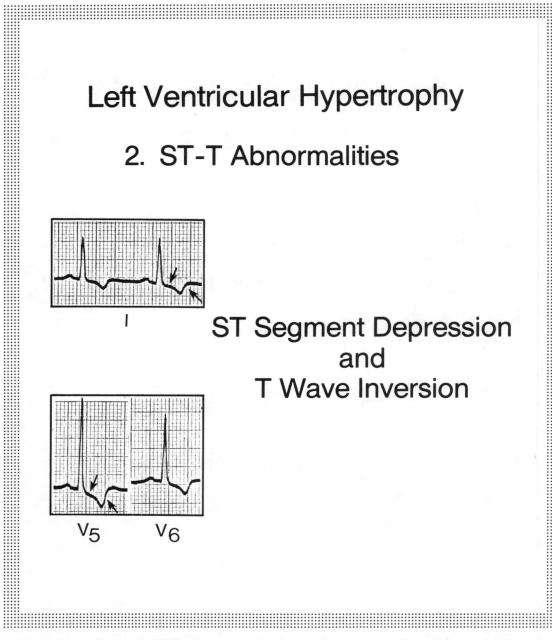

ST Segment Depression
and
T Wave Inversion

Ventricular repolarization (ST-T) abnormalities are frequently seen in left ventricular hypertrophy. The *QRS-T angle is wide*, with the T waves inverted. Note the asymmetry of the inverted T waves. There is a slow downstroke, followed by a rapid upstroke. *ST segment depression* is common.

Left Ventricular Hypertrophy
Principal Criteria
Review

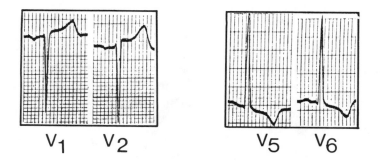

$$V_1 \quad\quad V_2 \quad\quad\quad\quad V_5 \quad\quad V_6$$

1. S_{V_1} or S_{V_2} + R_{V_5} or R_{V_6}

> 40 mm

2. ST-T Abnormalities

As the left ventricle hypertrophies, the mean QRS vector rotates more leftward and posteriorly. Left axis deviation may be seen in association with left ventricular hypertrophy, although
it is not a major electrocardiographic criterion. Ventricular repolarization (ST-T) abnormalities
are very common in left ventricular hypertrophy.

Note: The QRS magnitude criteria apply to *adults* since increased magnitude of the QRS
complex, without ST-T abnormalities may be seen in a *normal* youth.

Atrial Depolarization

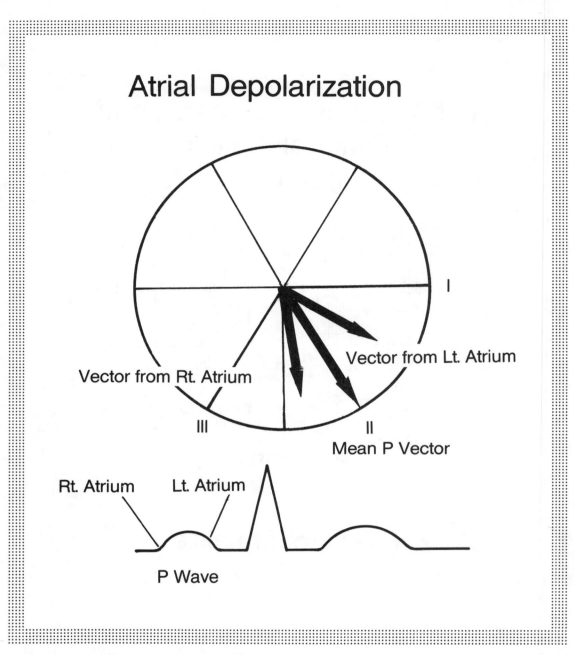

The mean P vector represents both atria. In order to understand atrial hypertrophy, we will study each atrium separately. The right atrium depolarizes first, represented by the initial portion of the P wave, followed by left atrial depolarization. The earlier right atrial vector is more rightward and anteriorly oriented compared with the left atrial vector, which is more leftward and posteriorly oriented.

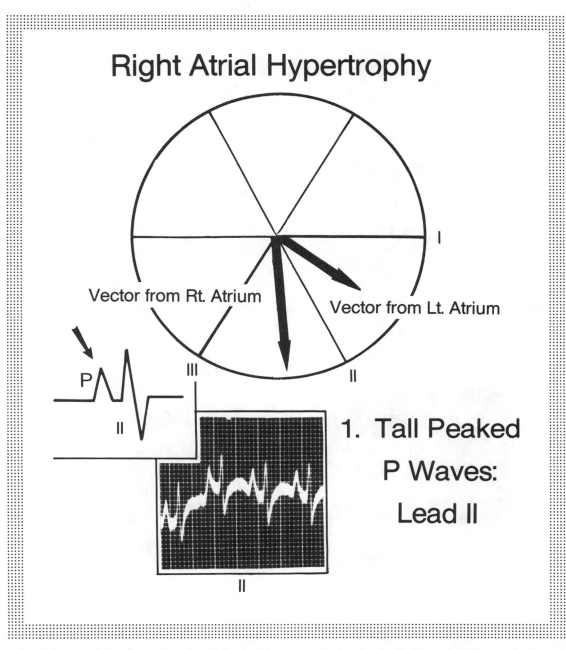

Right Atrial Hypertrophy

Vector from Rt. Atrium

Vector from Lt. Atrium

P

II

III

I

II

1. Tall Peaked
   P Waves:
   Lead II

II

In right atrial hypertrophy the right atrial vector, facing leads II, III and aVF, results in *tall early P waves* in these leads. The normal P wave is rarely more than 2 mm. in any lead and is rounded in contour, not peaked or notched.

Right Atrial Hypertrophy

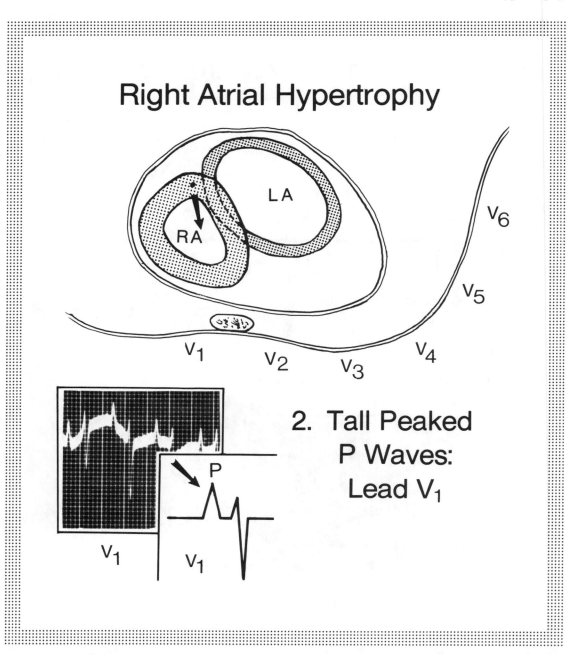

2. Tall Peaked P Waves: Lead V₁

Since the right atrial vector is *anterior*, facing lead V_1, the early part of the P wave, or even the entire P wave, may be *positive* and of great magnitude in lead V_1 in right atrial hypertrophy. This is in contrast to left atrial hypertrophy, in which the orientation of the left atrial vector is *posterior*, facing away from lead V_1, with deep *negative* P waves in lead V_1 (pp. 95-97).

Right Atrial Hypertrophy
Principal Criteria
Review

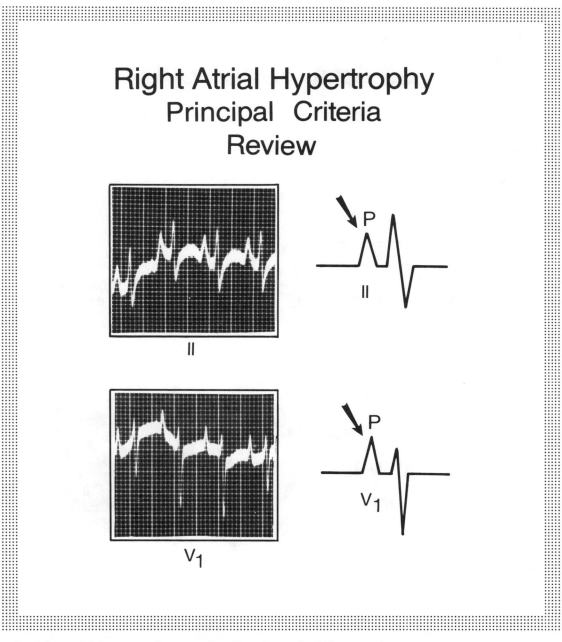

In right atrial hypertrophy we see tall early peaked P waves in

    Lead II, often also in leads III and aVF

    Lead V_1

Note: When evidence of right atrial hypertrophy is found in the electrocardiogram, it is good *presumptive evidence* of right *ventricular* hypertrophy, since right atrial hypertrophy rarely occurs alone.

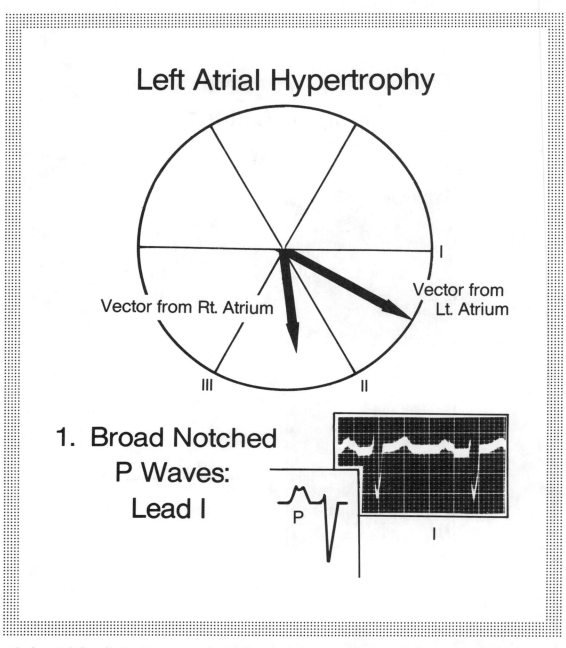

Left Atrial Hypertrophy

Vector from Rt. Atrium

Vector from
Lt. Atrium

I

III

II

1. Broad Notched P Waves: Lead I

P

I

Left atrial depolarization starts after right atrial depolarization. In left atrial hypertrophy, the left atrial vector, facing leads I and II, is delayed with broadening of the latter part of the P wave, forming a *notched P wave*. Since this was commonly seen in mitral valve disease, it became known as *P mitrale*.

Left Atrial Hypertrophy

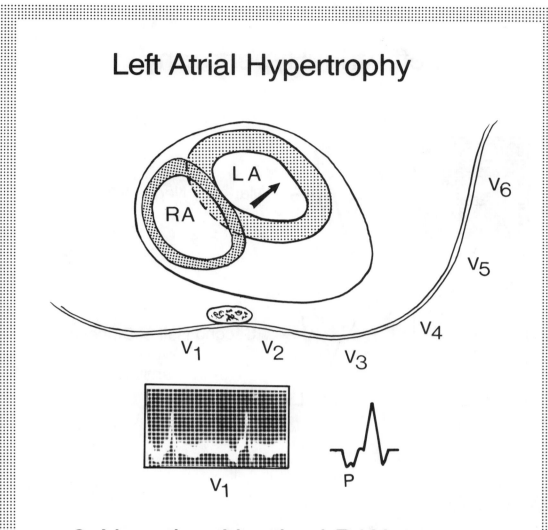

2. Negative, Notched P Waves: Lead V₁

Since the left atrial vector is *posterior*, facing away from lead V_1, the P wave in left atrial hypertrophy may be markedly *negative, broad and notched.* This is in contrast to the orientation of the right atrial vector, as already noted, which is anterior, facing lead V_1, with tall positive P waves in lead V_1 in right atrial hypertrophy.

Left Atrial Hypertrophy

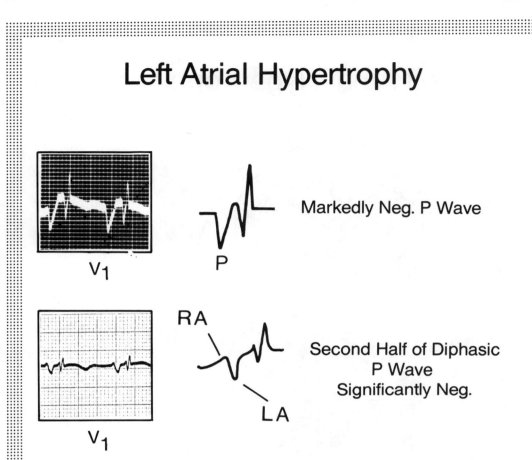

V₁   P   Markedly Neg. P Wave

RA
                              Second Half of Diphasic
                                      P Wave
                              Significantly Neg.
                              LA
V₁

Additional Types of P Wave Configurations in Lead V₁, Associated with Left Atrial Hypertrophy

In addition to the negative, broad and notched P wave seen on the previous page, two additional types of P waves may be seen in lead V₁ in association with left atrial hypertrophy. The common characteristic is that *either the entire P wave or the second part is abnormally negative.*

Left Atrial Hypertrophy
Principal Criteria
Review

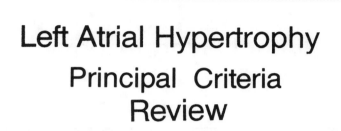

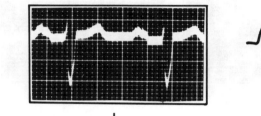

I

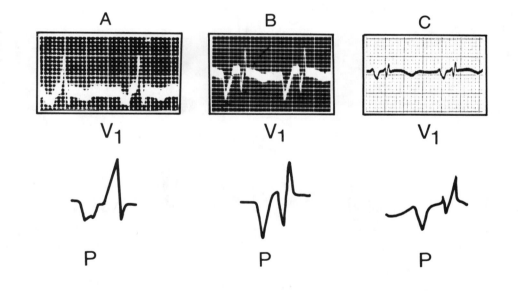

In left atrial hypertrophy the following types of P waves may be seen:

Lead I—Broad, notched P waves

Lead V_1—Negative P waves of increased magnitude:

  A. Broad and notched

  B. Entirely negative

  C. Second part of diphasic P wave, markedly negative

Biatrial Hypertrophy

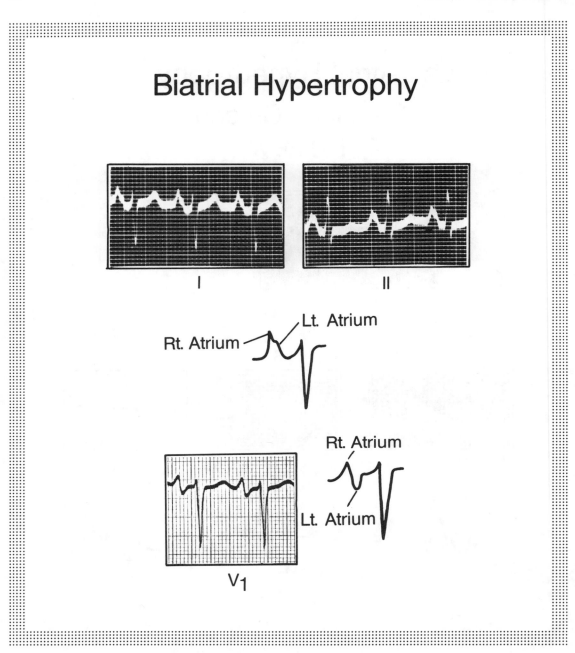

Biatrial hypertrophy has features of both right and left atrial hypertrophy. In leads I and II we have the early peaking of the P wave of right atrial hypertrophy and the notching of left atrial hypertrophy. In lead V_1 we see the prominent first half of the diphasic P wave of right atrial hypertrophy and the significantly negative second half, representing left atrial hypertrophy.

Practice
ECG Analysis

Practice
ECG Analysis

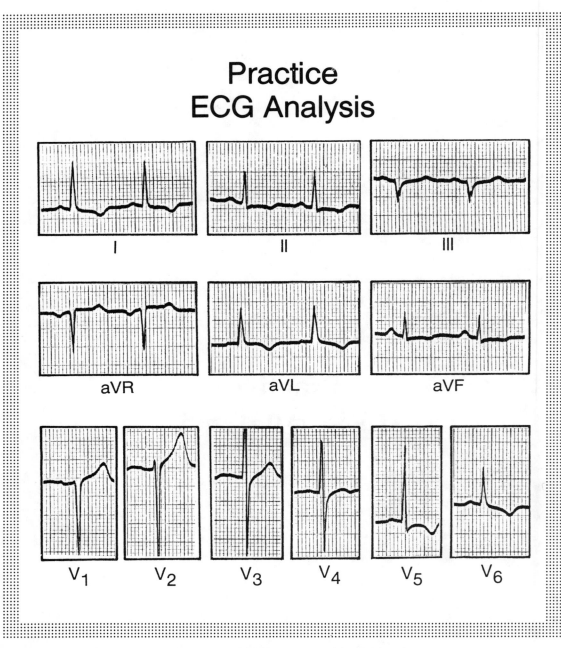

The patient is a 69 year old woman with a history of high blood pressure.

Analysis:

ECG ANALYSIS

1. Rhythm and Rate
   Rhythm: Sinus Rhythm
   Rate: 80/min.
   PR Interval: 0.16 sec.
2. QRS Complex
   Duration: 0.08 sec.
   Axis: +15°
   $S_{V_2} + R_{V_5} = 45$ mm.
3. Ventricular Repolarization
   ST Segment: Depressed in leads II, aVF and V_5
   T Wave: T waves inverted in leads I, II, aVF, V_5 and V_6
      QRS-T angle very wide
4. QT Interval: 0.38 sec.

Impression and Comment

Left Ventricular Hypertrophy
Ventricular Repolarization (ST-T) Abnormalities

Increased magnitude of the ventricular deflections (QRS complexes) is the major electrocardiographic criterion for left ventricular hypertrophy, seen best in the precordial leads, V_1 to V_6. The diagnosis of left ventricular hypertrophy should not be made without evidence of increased magnitude. Ventricular repolarization (ST-T) abnormalities usually accompany left ventricular hypertrophy, although ischemia of the myocardium may additionally contribute.

Practice
ECG Analysis

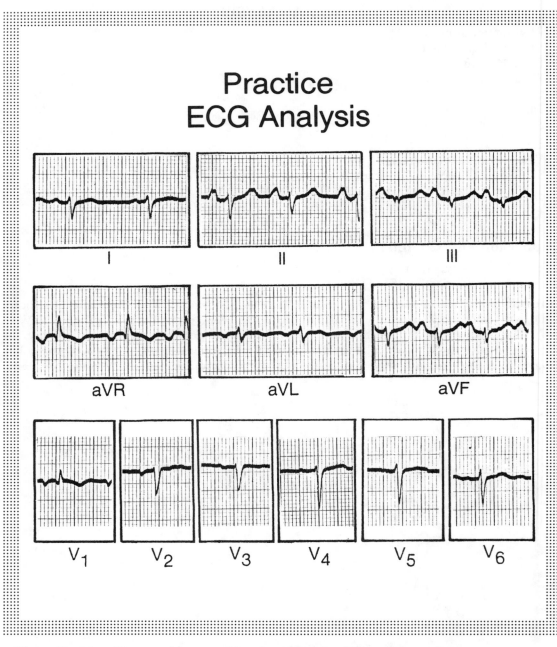

The patient is a 73 year old man with a long history of chronic lung disease.

Analysis:

ECG ANALYSIS

1. Rhythm and Rate
   Rhythm: Sinus Rhythm
   Rate: 95/min.
   PR Interval: 0.18 sec.
   Prominent P waves, leads II, III and aVF
2. QRS Complex
   Duration: 0.08 sec.
   Axis: −135° (extreme right axis deviation)
   R wave in lead V_1 is the main ventricular deflection
3. Ventricular Repolarization
   ST Segment: Neither significantly elevated nor depressed
   T Wave: Abnormally wide QRS-T angle
4. QT Interval: 0.35 sec.

Impression and Comment

Right Ventricular Hypertrophy
Ventricular Repolarization Abnormalities

The extreme right axis deviation (−135°) and the predominant R wave in lead V_1, as well as the abnormally wide QRS-T angle, are the important criteria. The prominent P waves in leads II, III and aVF represent the accompanying right atrial hypertrophy. This patient, who had been smoking for more than 50 years, was suffering from bronchitis, emphysema and heart failure.

Chapter 3

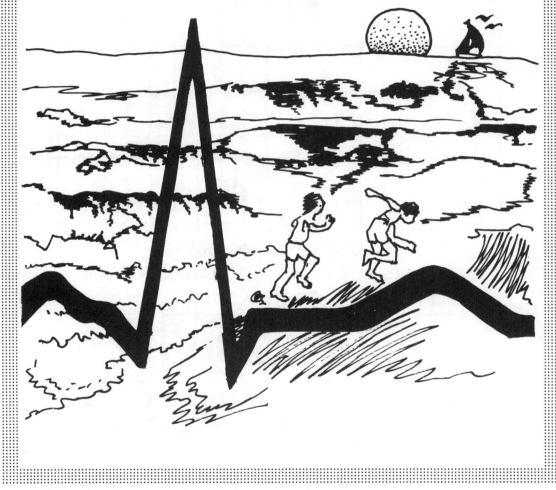

Ventricular Repolarization (ST-T) Alterations

Ventricular *repolarization* is a longer process and consumes more energy than *depolarization*. It is, therefore, much more prone to alterations and abnormalities; hence the multiple causes of ST-T abnormalities. On the other hand, not every ST segment or T wave that appears abnormal at first is actually abnormal. This can be observed in the *early repolarization* and *juvenile* patterns, to be seen shortly. We have actually started studying ventricular repolarization in the first two chapters.

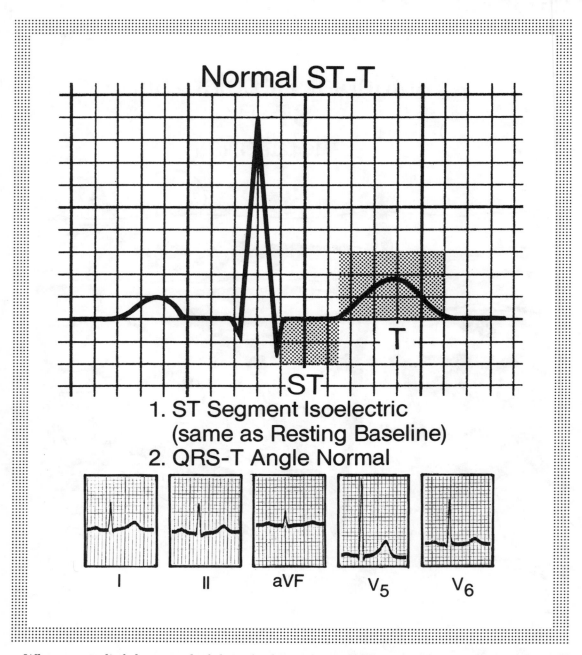

When we studied the normal adult in the first chapter, we found that often the QRS-T angle is less than 45° and rarely wider than 60°. *For the QRS-T angle to be normally narrow, the T wave should have the same orientation as the QRS complex in leads I, II, aVF, V_5 and V_6.*

The ST segment is normally *isoelectric, same as the resting baseline, neither elevated nor depressed.* It may, however, slope upward toward a relatively tall T wave.

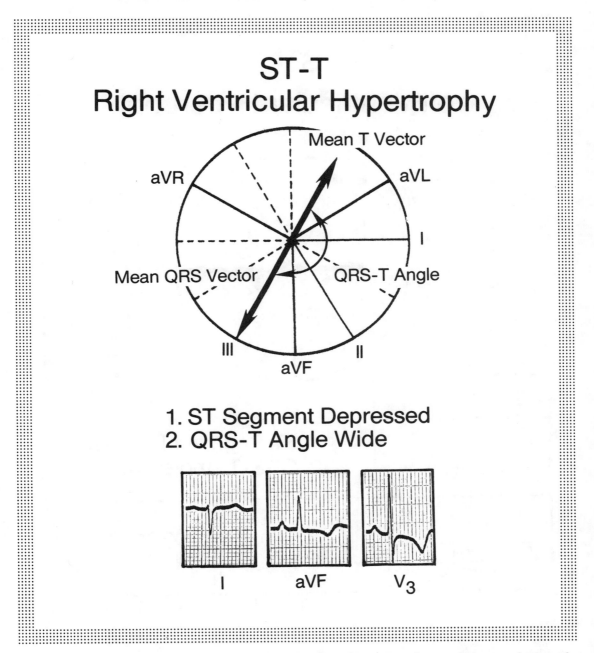

ST-T
Right Ventricular Hypertrophy

1. ST Segment Depressed
2. QRS-T Angle Wide

In the second chapter we found that ventricular repolarization abnormalities are frequently seen in right ventricular hypertrophy. In the above electrocardiogram, note the wide QRS-T angle. The QRS complexes and T waves are opposite in orientation. Where the QRS complex is positive, the T wave is negative, and where the QRS complex is negative, the T wave is positive. *The QRS-T angle is, therefore, extremely wide, 180°.* ST segment depression is seen in lead V₃.

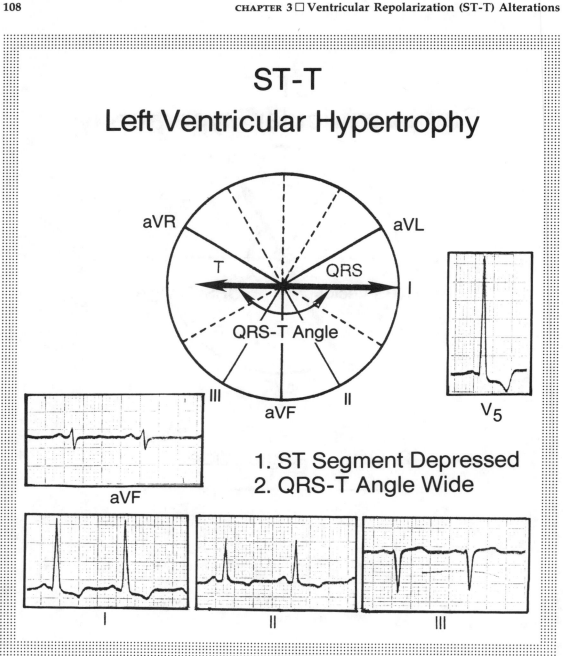

ST-T
Left Ventricular Hypertrophy

1. ST Segment Depressed
2. QRS-T Angle Wide

As they do in right ventricular hypertrophy, ventricular repolarization abnormalities generally accompany left ventricular hypertrophy. Note the very wide QRS-T angle above. Where the QRS complex is positive, the T wave is negative, and where the QRS complex is negative, the T wave is positive. They share the transition at lead aVF. ST segment depression is seen in leads I and V_5.

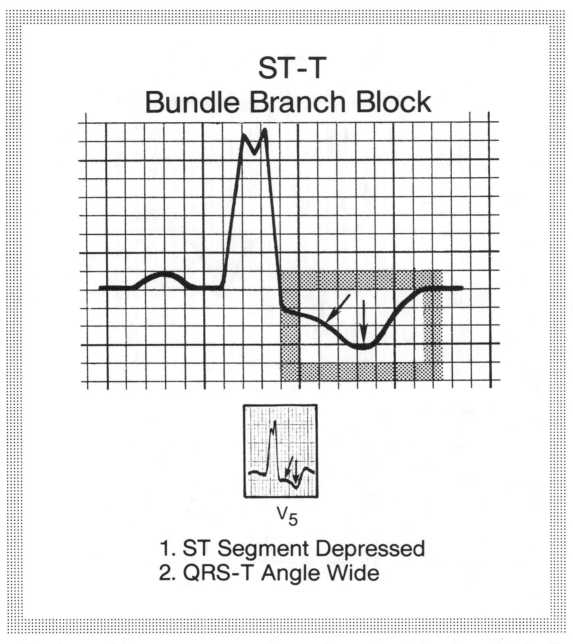

ST-T
Bundle Branch Block

V₅

1. ST Segment Depressed
2. QRS-T Angle Wide

This electrocardiogram represents an intraventricular conduction disturbance (left bundle branch block), to be studied in Chapter 5. For the present, note the abnormal width of the QRS complex and the repolarization abnormalities. When depolarization is abnormal, as seen above, repolarization is also abnormal.

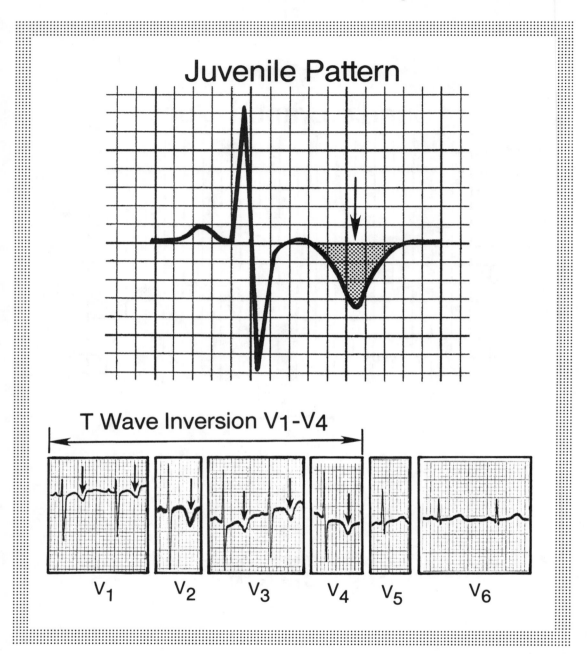

In youth the mean T vector is frequently to the left, inferior and posterior, inscribing T waves across the chest that are negative in leads V_1, V_2, V_3 and often V_4. This is known as the *juvenile pattern.* This pattern is not infrequently seen in normal healthy young patients well into the third decade of life. This emphasizes that the electrocardiogram should not be read without knowing the age of the patient or without knowledge of pertinent clinical information.

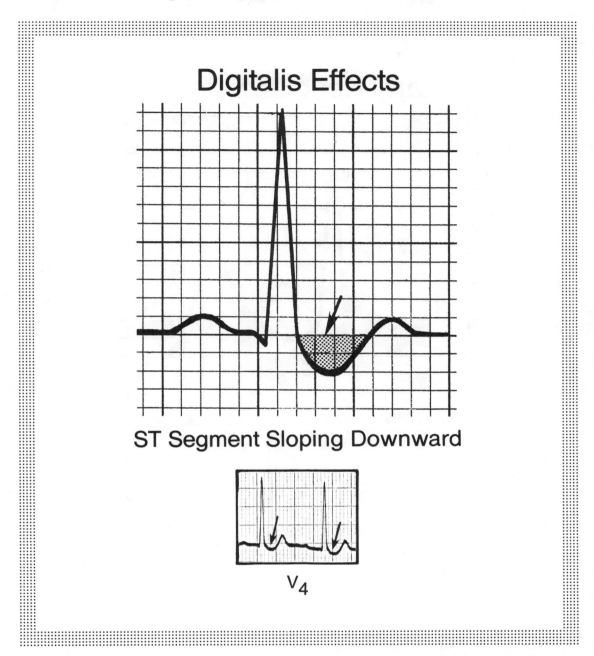

Digitalis Effects

ST Segment Sloping Downward

V₄

Digitalis has long been known for its effects on ventricular repolarization. The "classic" changes of the ST segment caused by digitalis have been described as a *paintbrush inscription* (as if you were painting the ST segment with gradual widening of the brush stroke), or a *fist-like depression* of the ST segment (as if you were placing a fist in the ST segment and depressing it), or *scooping* of the ST segment. These alterations are known as "digitalis effects."

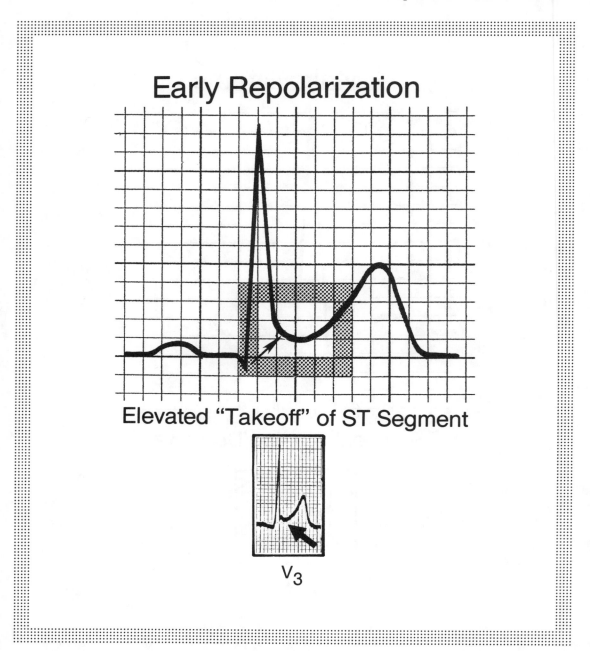

Early Repolarization

Elevated "Takeoff" of ST Segment

V₃

A common repolarization variant, seen in normal young adults, is ST segment displacement, usually associated with tall or deep T waves. This pattern has been known as *early repolarization* and is not considered abnormal. Note the elevation of the QRS-ST junction (J point). The electrocardiogram is normal in all other aspects. Of importance is the need to distinguish early repolarization from the more ominous causes of ST segment displacement, such as pericarditis and myocardial infarction.

Pericarditis

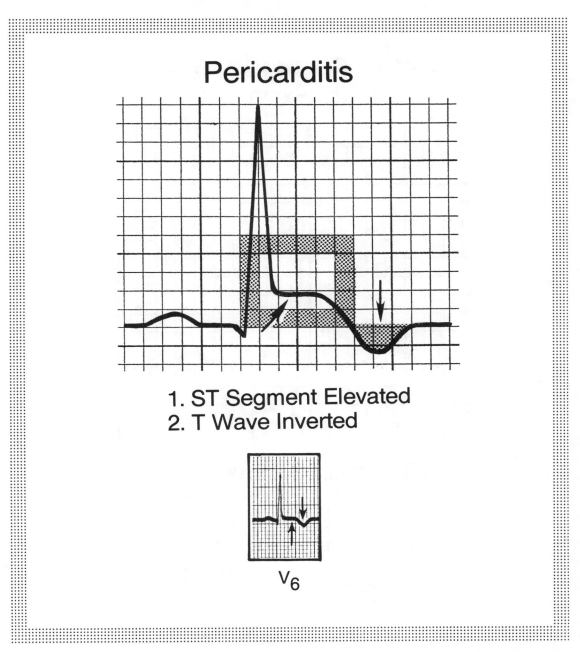

1. ST Segment Elevated
2. T Wave Inverted

V_6

Ventricular repolarization abnormalities are common in patients with *pericarditis*. Often both the ST segment and the T wave are involved. Do not confuse this abnormal, changing and evolving pattern with early repolarization found in healthy young patients. Clinical correlation must be stressed, since the electrocardiographic changes seen above may not be distinguishable from those of a patient with an acute myocardial infarction.

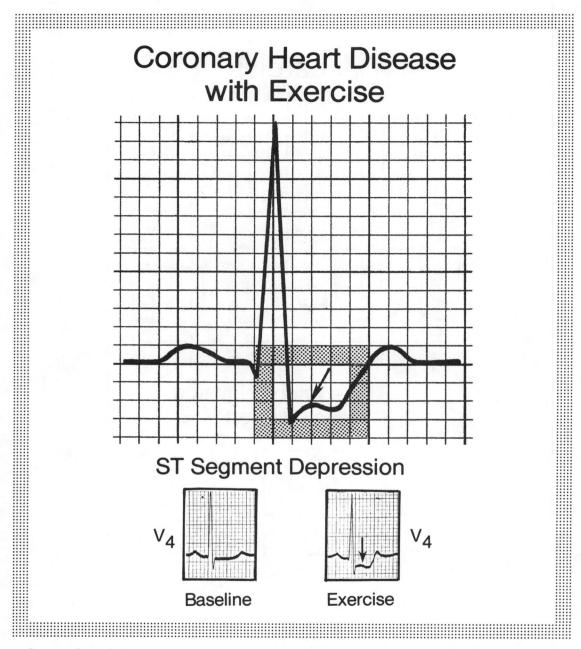

Coronary Heart Disease with Exercise

ST Segment Depression

V4   V4

Baseline   Exercise

Coronary heart disease is a major cause of ventricular repolarization abnormalities. The marked depression, with exercise, of the ST segment recorded above occurred in a patient with a history of angina pectoris. Some patients with a typical history of angina pectoris have an electrocardiogram with normal ventricular repolarization *at rest*. Quite often, utilizing the patient's normal activity, such as taking a walk, yields important information in the initial evaluation.

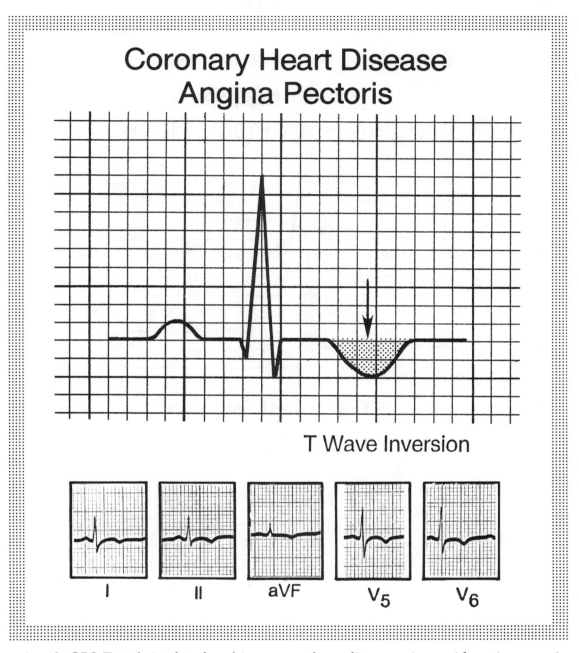

Coronary Heart Disease
Angina Pectoris

T Wave Inversion

I   II   aVF   V₅   V₆

A wide QRS-T angle is often found in coronary heart disease patients with angina pectoris. Note that the QRS complexes and T waves are opposite in orientation. The term *ischemia* is frequently applied to this wide QRS-T angle. When the cause is not known, this abnormality is labeled *nonspecific*.

Variant Angina Pectoris
(Angina Pectoris at Rest)

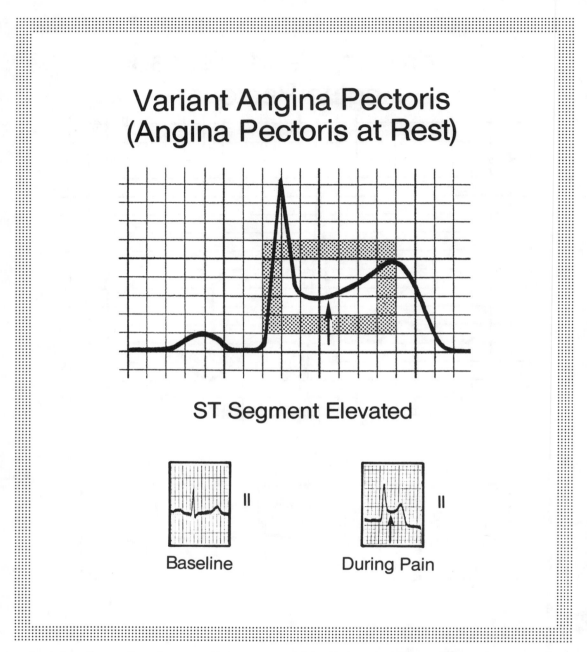

ST Segment Elevated

Baseline   During Pain

A variant form of angina pectoris was reported by Prinzmetal. The striking elevation of the ST segment in lead II occurred in a patient with a history of angina pectoris, principally *at rest*. This marked ST segment elevation resembles that of the hyperacute phase of myocardial infarction (next chapter) but lasts only a few minutes. This disorder is commonly caused by spasm of the coronary arteries.

Ventricular Aneurysm

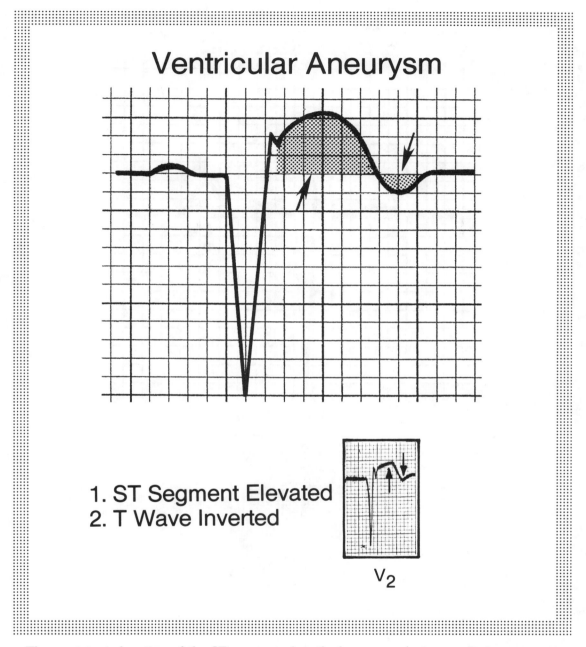

1. ST Segment Elevated
2. T Wave Inverted

V_2

The persistent elevation of the ST segment, described as a *monophasic curve of injury,* represents a ventricular aneurysm, an outpouching of a section of scarred ventricular myocardium. The electrocardiogram resembles that of an acute myocardial infarction (next chapter). In order to exclude an acute myocardial infarction, always ask for comparison electrocardiograms.

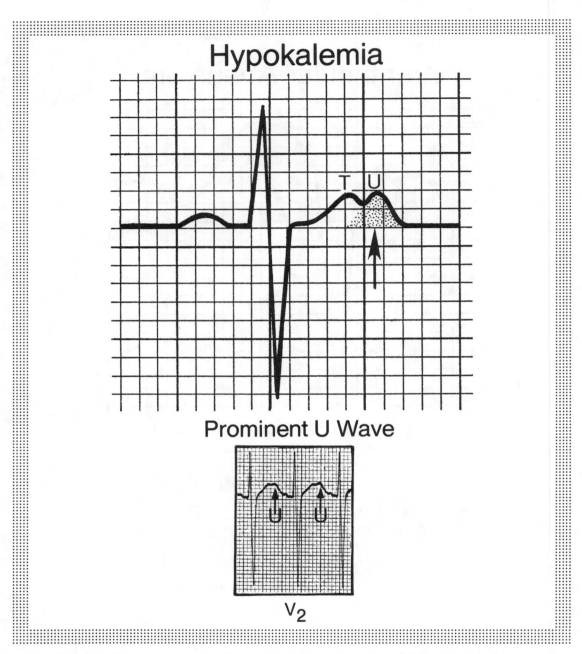

Hypokalemia

Prominent U Wave

V₂

Hypokalemia (low potassium level) may produce striking electrocardiographic abnormalities, such as depression of the ST segment, lowering and flattening of the T wave and appearance of a *U wave*. The U wave is a wave that follows the T wave and has frequently been associated with hypokalemia, although it may be found normally. During correction of the hypokalemia, close electrocardiographic follow-up of this patient revealed a T wave that gradually became taller and a U wave that gradually disappeared.

U Wave

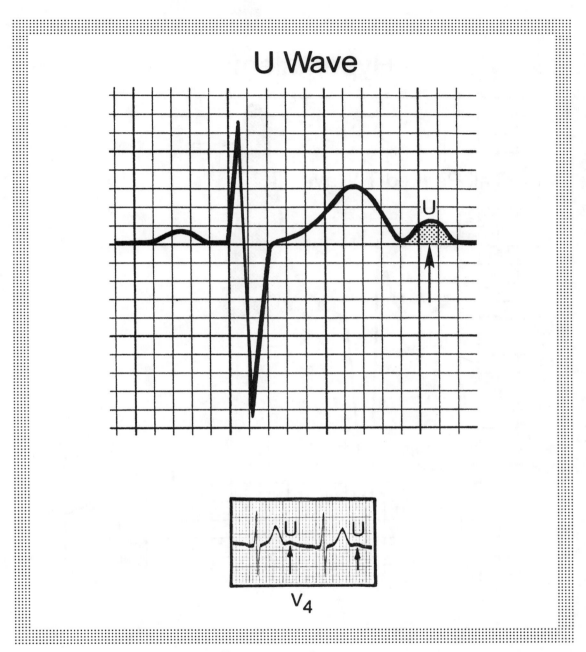

Although the U wave, which follows the T wave, has been associated with hypokalemia (which causes its accentuation), it may be found normally. It is often seen best in the mid-precordial leads (V_3 and V_4, as above), and it has the same orientation as the T wave.

Hyperkalemia

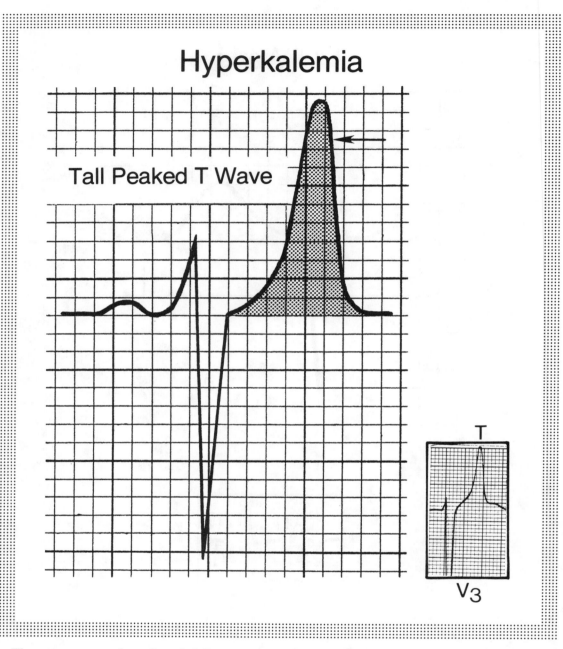

The appearance of *a tall, peaked T wave* is a manifestation of hyperkalemia (high potassium level). With increasingly high blood levels of potassium, the PR interval is prolonged, with a widening QRS interval. In more extreme cases of hyperkalemia, the P waves become flatter and the QRS complexes continue to widen. Ventricular fibrillation may then ensue if the level of potassium continues to rise.

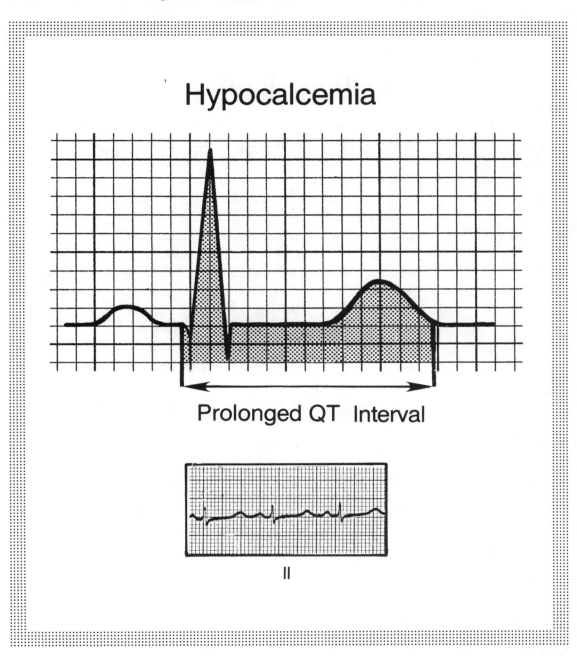

Hypocalcemia

Prolonged QT Interval

II

The QT interval may be *markedly prolonged* in a patient with hypocalcemia (low calcium level). This patient's heart rate is 84 per minute. At this rate the QT interval should be approximately 0.35 sec. rather than 0.52 sec., as seen here. Review (p. 54) the relationship between the QT interval and the heart rate.

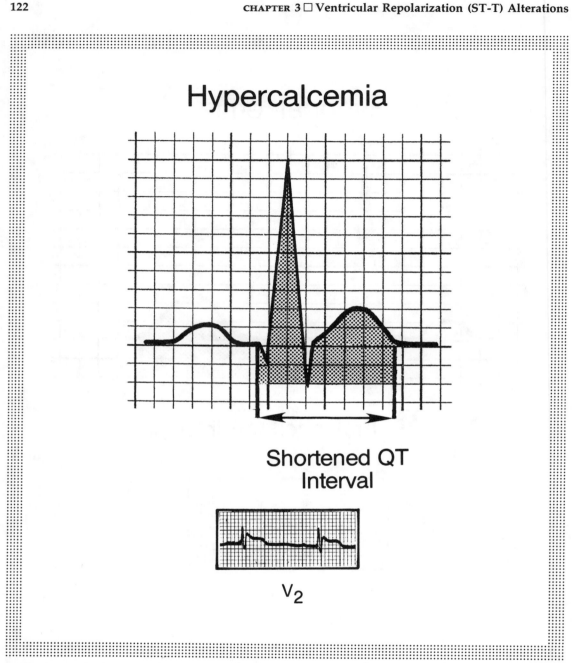

Hypercalcemia

Shortened QT
Interval

V$_2$

Hypercalcemia (high calcium level) is often represented electrocardiographically by a *short QT interval*. There is an inverse relationship between the QT interval and the level of serum calcium.

Practice
ECG Analysis

Practice
ECG Analysis

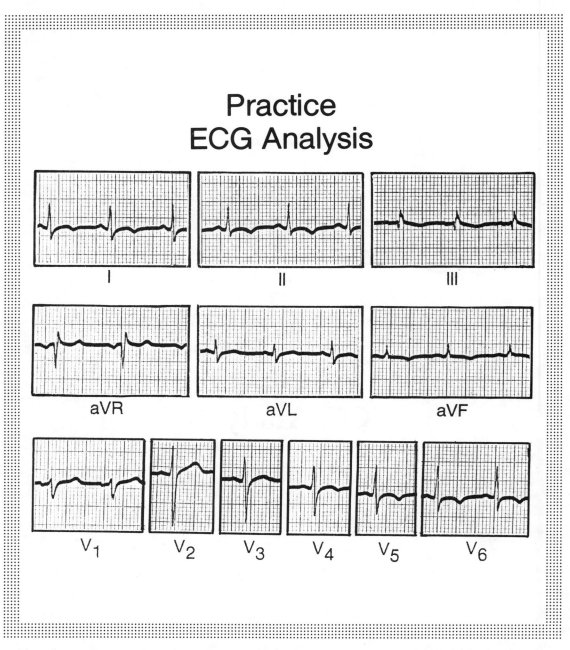

The patient is a 60 year old man with a history of stable angina pectoris, responsive to treatment with nitroglycerine.

Analysis:

ECG ANALYSIS

1. Rhythm and Rate
   Rhythm: Sinus Rhythm
   Rate: 90/min.
   PR Interval: 0.14 sec.
2. QRS Complex
   Duration: 0.08 sec.
   Axis: $+60°$
3. Ventricular Repolarization
   ST Segment: Not significantly elevated or depressed
T Wave: Inverted in leads I, II, III, aVF, V_4 to V_6
   QRS-T angle very wide
4. QT Interval: 0.36 sec.

Impression and Comment

Ventricular Repolarization Abnormalities
Compatible with Coronary Heart Disease

A wide QRS-T angle is frequently found in coronary heart disease patients with angina pectoris. Note that the QRS complexes and T waves are opposite in orientation. The term *ischemia* is often applied to this wide QRS-T angle. Evaluation of this patient revealed significant coronary heart disease with myocardial ischemia. When the cause is not known, this abnormality is labeled *nonspecific.*

Practice
ECG Analysis

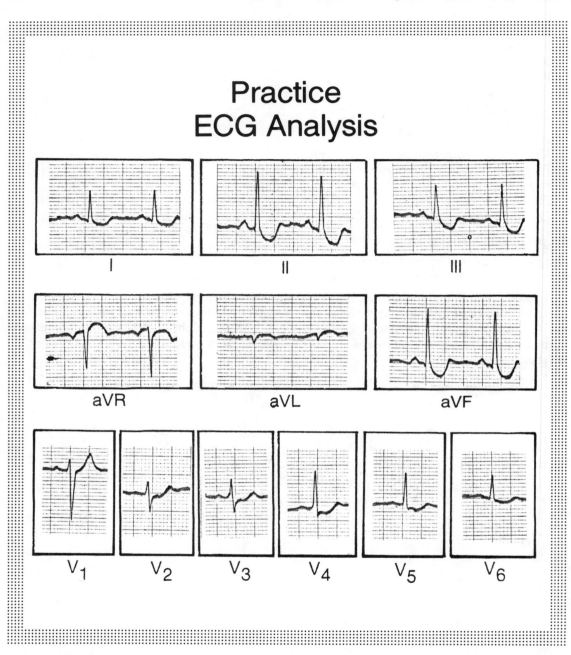

The patient is a 75 year old woman with congestive heart failure, for which she is taking digitalis and diuretics.

Analysis:

ECG ANALYSIS

1. Rhythm and Rate
   Rhythm: Sinus Rhythm
   Rate: 85 min.
   PR Interval: 0.16 sec.
2. QRS Complex
   Duration: 0.08 sec.
   Axis: $+65°$
3. Ventricular Repolarization
   ST Segment: Rounded ST segments, depressed in leads I, II, III, aVF and V_6, elevated in lead
   aVR. ST segment also depressed in leads V_2 to V_5
   T Wave: Flat or low in leads I, II, III, aVF, V_5 and V_6, inverted in aVL; however, the QRS-
   T angle is not wide.
4. QT Interval: 0.34 sec.

Impression and Comment

Ventricular Repolarization Alterations
Compatible with Digitalis Effects and Myocardial Ischemia

The paintbrush inscription of the ST segments, seen especially well in leads II, III and aVF, as well as the lowering and flattening of the T waves, is commonly seen as a result of "digitalis effects." The depressed origin or "take-off" of the ST segments (J point) in leads V_2, V_3, V_4 and V_5, present before the patient started taking digitalis, is compatible with the myocardial ischemia from her known coronary heart disease

Practice
ECG Analysis

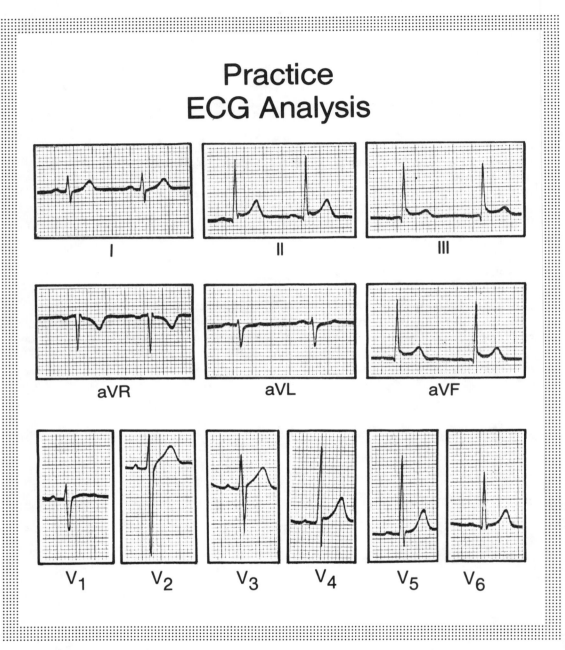

The patient is a healthy 18 year old student.

Analysis:

ECG ANALYSIS

1. Rhythm and Rate
   Rhythm: Sinus Rhythm
   Rate: 75 / min.
   PR Interval: 0.14 sec.
2. QRS Complex
   Duration: 0.08 sec.
   Axis: $+85°$
3. Ventricular Repolarization
   ST Segment: Elevated origin of the ST segment, especially well seen in leads II, III, aVF, V_4 and V_5
   T Wave: QRS-T angle normal
4. QT Interval: 0.35 sec.

Impression and Comment

Normal Electrocardiogram with Early Repolarization

Early repolarization is a common variant seen in normal young adults. The electrocardiogram is normal in all other respects. Of importance is the need to distinguish early repolarization from the more ominous causes of ST segment displacement, such as pericarditis or myocardial infarction.

Chapter 4

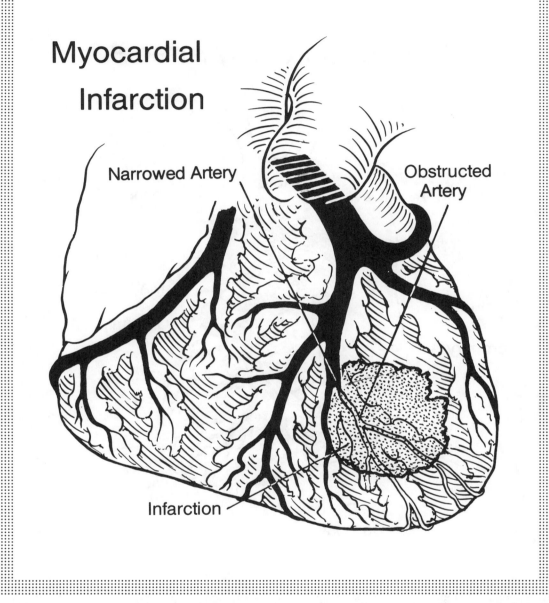

Myocardial Infarction

Narrowed Artery

Obstructed Artery

Infarction

When the blood supply to an area of the heart is obstructed, a section of heart muscle may die. This is known as infarction of the heart muscle or *myocardial infarction.*

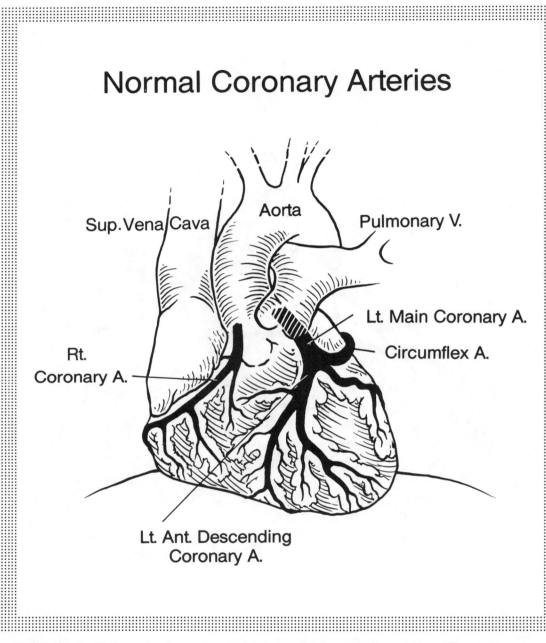

Normal Coronary Arteries

Sup.Vena Cava   Aorta   Pulmonary V.

Rt. Coronary A.

Lt. Main Coronary A.

Circumflex A.

Lt. Ant. Descending Coronary A.

Blood is supplied to the heart by the right and left coronary arteries. The right coronary artery remains a major trunk throughout its length, whereas the left coronary artery, after a short main stem, divides into the left anterior descending and circumflex arteries.

Left Ventricle

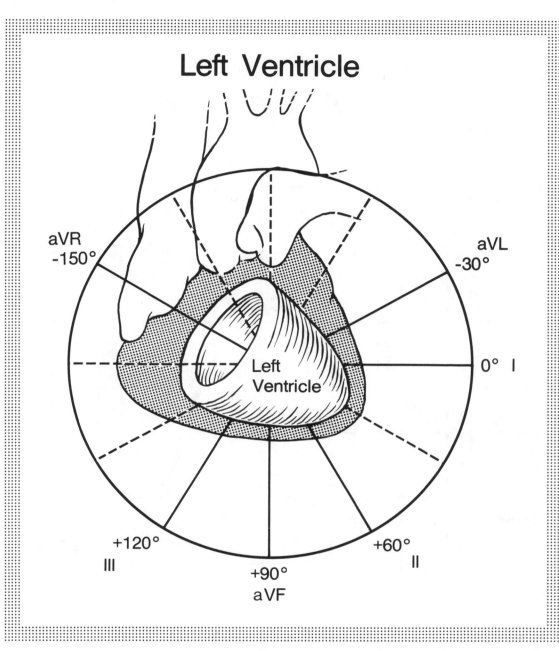

The left ventricle is the chamber of the heart most frequently associated with myocardial infarction. It will, therefore, be the subject of study in this chapter.

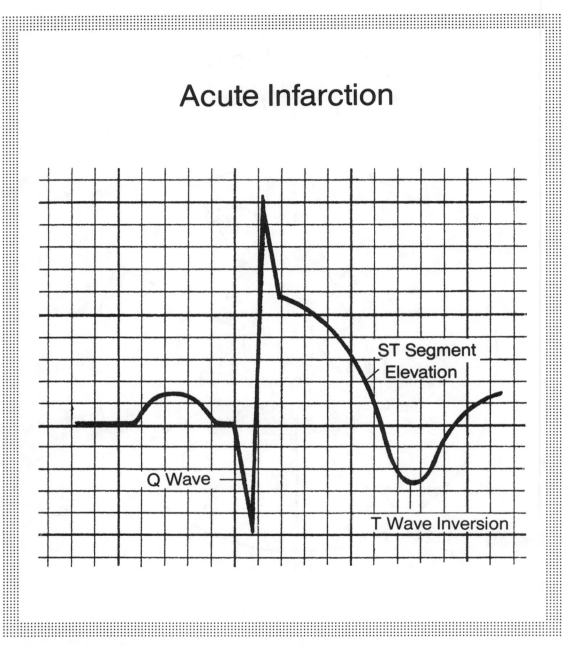

The classic electrocardiographic changes encountered in acute myocardial infarction are
 1. *The Q wave,*
 2. *ST segment elevation and*
 3. *T wave inversion.*

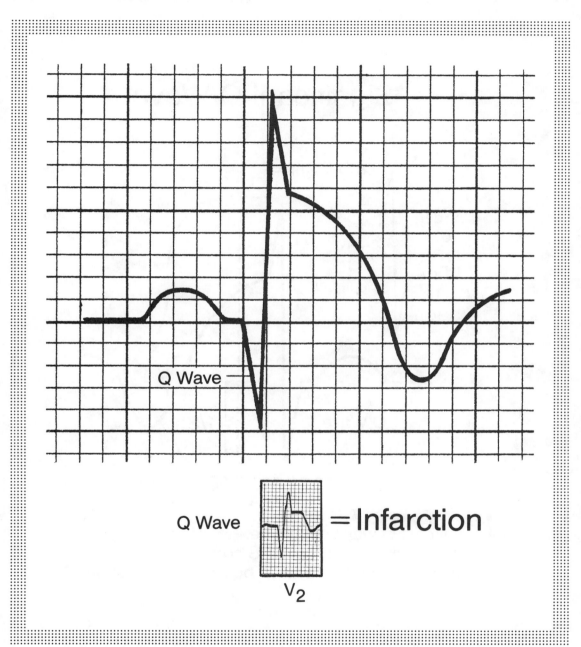

Q Wave

Q Wave = Infarction

V₂

The Q wave, the first negative deflection of the QRS complex following the P wave, is *the electrocardiographic manifestation of myocardial infarction.* The Q wave must, however, be *significant*, since in normal patients small Q waves are frequently seen in various leads (I, aVL, V_5, V_6).

Significant Q Wave

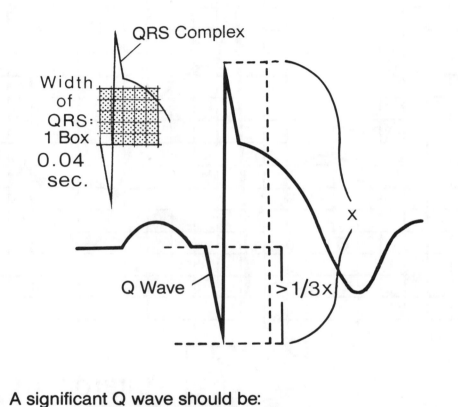

A significant Q wave should be:
1. One-third height of QRS complex
2. 0.04 second (one small box wide) in duration

The *significant Q wave* is at least *one third the height of the QRS complex* and *0.04 second in duration (1 small box wide)*. Lead aVR is the exception, since a large Q wave is normal.

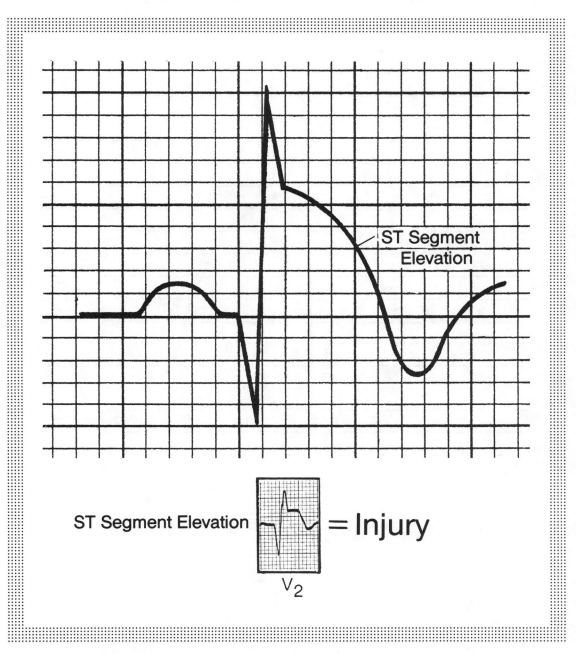

The elevated ST segment seen in acute myocardial infarction is known as the *current of injury.* Because of its appearance, it is sometimes referred to as the *monophasic curve of injury.*

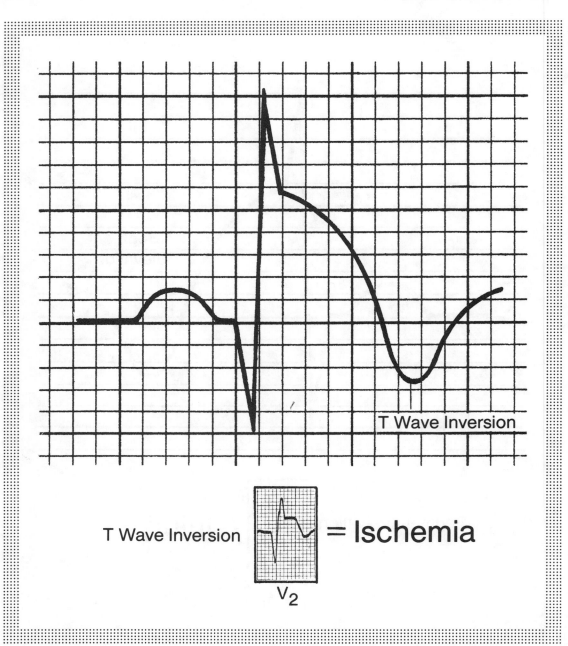

T Wave Inversion

T Wave Inversion = Ischemia

V_2

Inverted T waves are often seen in myocardial infarction, signifying *ischemia* (diminished blood supply). As already noted, inverted T waves, forming a wide QRS-T angle, are a frequent finding in electrocardiography.

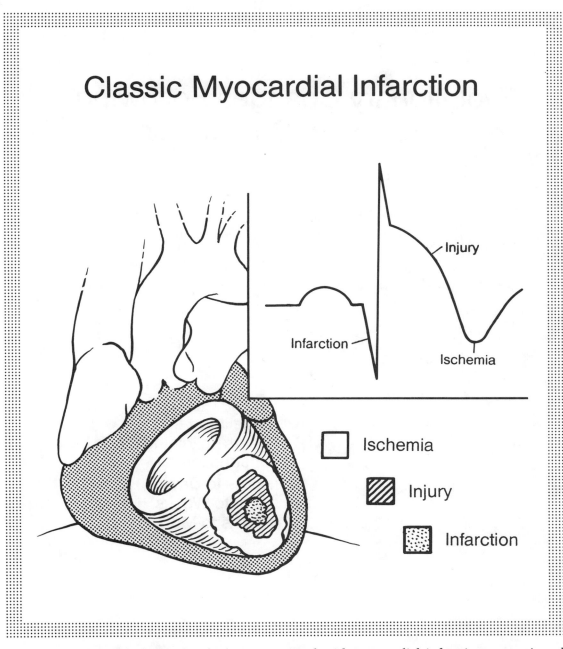

Classic Myocardial Infarction

Injury

Infarction

Ischemia

☐ Ischemia

▨ Injury

▦ Infarction

The *classic* electrocardiographic findings associated with myocardial infarction are reviewed above. Any of the three, however, may be found alone. The accompanying diagram shows an infarcted zone surrounded by zones of injury and ischemia.

Evolutionary Changes Following Blood Flow Obstruction

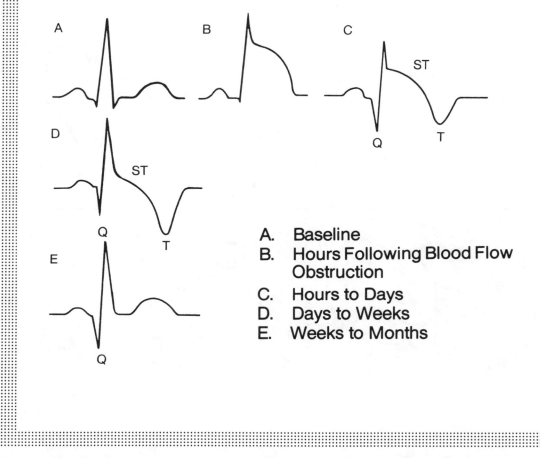

A. Baseline
B. Hours Following Blood Flow
    Obstruction
C. Hours to Days
D. Days to Weeks
E. Weeks to Months

Note that the ST segment elevation occurs prior to the formation of the Q wave. During these early hours, interventions are often undertaken to reverse the process. As time passes the Q wave forms, the ST segment is less elevated and the T wave inverts. The final outcome varies greatly, depending on the amount of myocardial damage.

Areas of Infarction
(Left Ventricle)

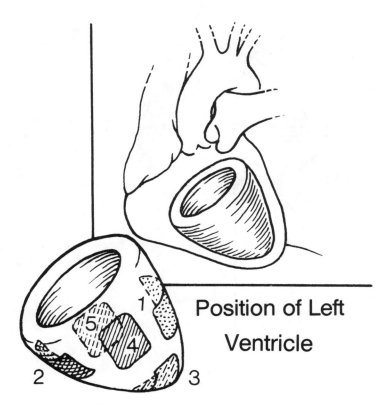

Position of Left

Ventricle

The illustration shows the division of the left ventricle into regions where infarction may occur. These regions are

1. Lateral
2. Diaphragmatic or Inferior
3. Apical
4. Anterior
5. Posterior.

Lateral Infarction

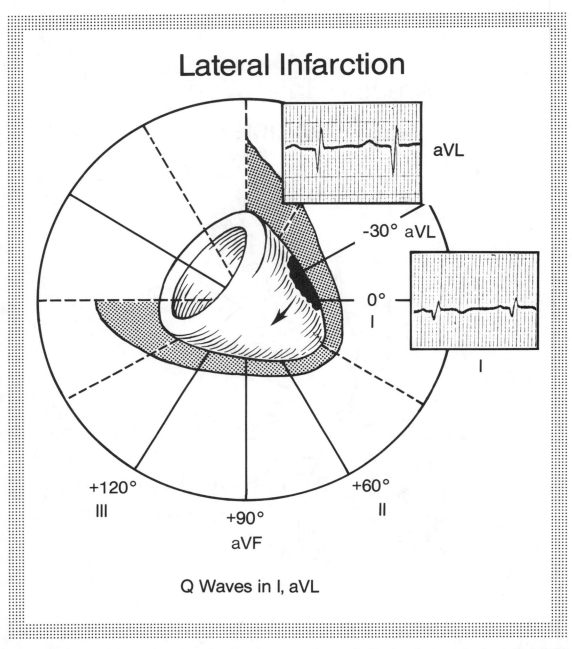

Q Waves in I, aVL

In *lateral* myocardial infarction, the initial vector of ventricular depolarization, the initial QRS vector (arrow), moves *away* from the infarcted area, away from leads I and aVL, hence the formation of significant Q waves in these leads. *The Q wave represents initial vectorial forces moving away from the electrode at the point of recording.*

Lateral Infarction

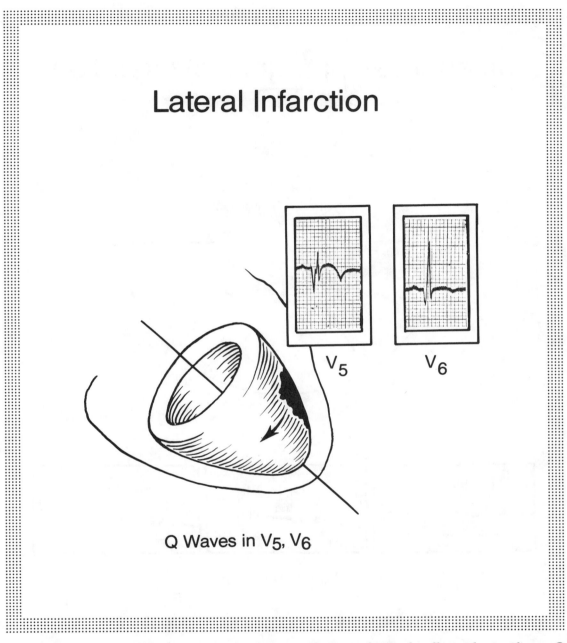

V_5 V_6

Q Waves in V_5, V_6

Lateral myocardial infarction may also be seen electrocardiographically with significant Q waves in the lateral precordial leads, V_5 and V_6. The initial QRS vector (arrow) moves away from leads V_5 and V_6.

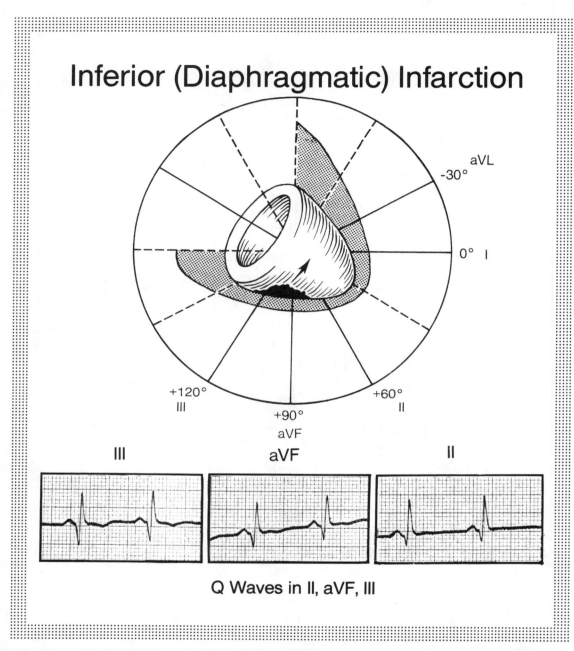

Inferior (Diaphragmatic) Infarction

Q Waves in II, aVF, III

In *inferior (diaphragmatic)* myocardial infarction, the initial vector of ventricular depolarization moves away from the diaphragmatic area, away from leads II, aVF and III. Significant Q waves are, thereby, formed in these leads.

Apical Infarction

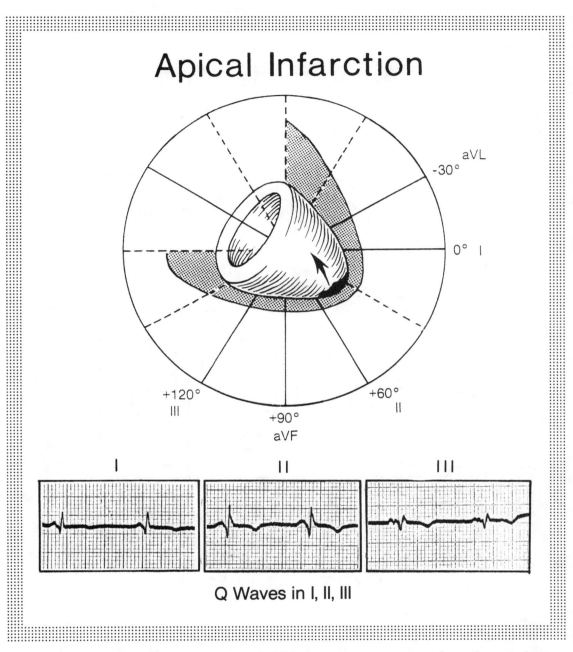

Q Waves in I, II, III

In *apical* myocardial infarction, the initial QRS vector, pointing away from the apical myocardium and from leads I, II and III, produces Q waves in all three leads. The question arises: Did one myocardial infarction produce these abnormalities, or are they the result of more than one infarction at different times? Serial electrocardiograms are vital in this determination.

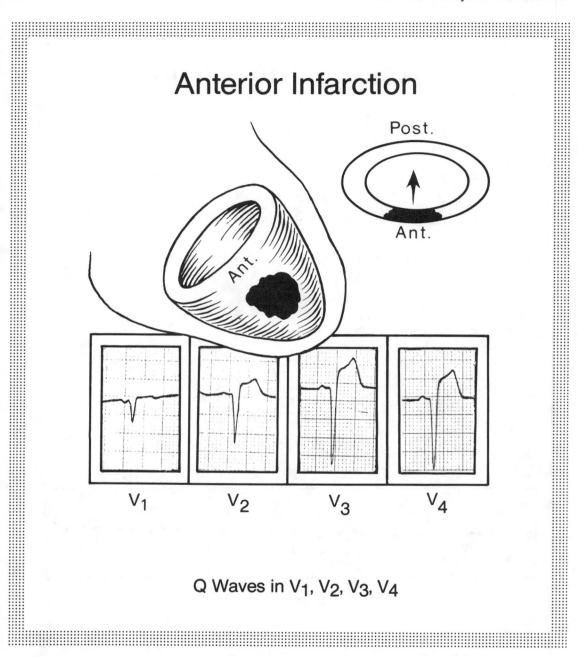

Anterior Infarction

Q Waves in V₁, V₂, V₃, V₄

In *anterior* or *anteroseptal* myocardial infarction, the initial QRS vector (arrow) moves away from the anterior surface and away from the anterior chest leads; hence the occurrence of significant Q waves in these leads.

Posterior Infarction

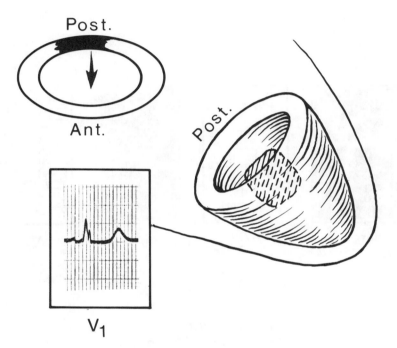

Prominent or Predominant R Wave in V₁

In *posterior* myocardial infarction, the initial QRS vector (arrow) moves away from the posterior wall of the left ventricle, located posteriorly and to the left. This initial vector, therefore, moves anteriorly and to the right, toward lead V_1, inscribing a positive deflection, a *predominant R wave in lead V_1*. This R wave in posterior myocardial infarction represents the same phenomenon as the Q wave in anterior myocardial infarction.

Infarction Without Q Waves

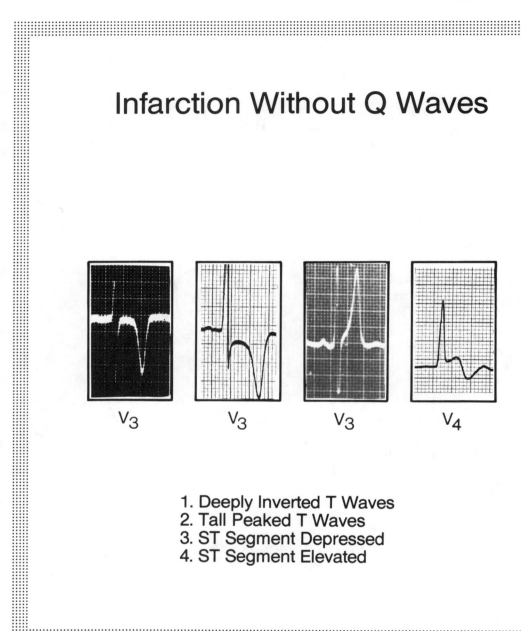

V₃   V₃   V₃   V₄

1. Deeply Inverted T Waves
2. Tall Peaked T Waves
3. ST Segment Depressed
4. ST Segment Elevated

Clinical evidence of infarction of the heart is frequently encountered without Q waves on the electrocardiogram. Although it may be misleading, the term *subendocardial* infarction has been used in this context. The clinical picture of infarction should be quite clear before an electrocardiogram is labeled subendocardial infarction, since these repolarization abnormalities, although striking, may be nonspecific. Similar findings may occur during angina pectoris (negative T waves) and electrolyte imbalance (tall, peaked T waves).

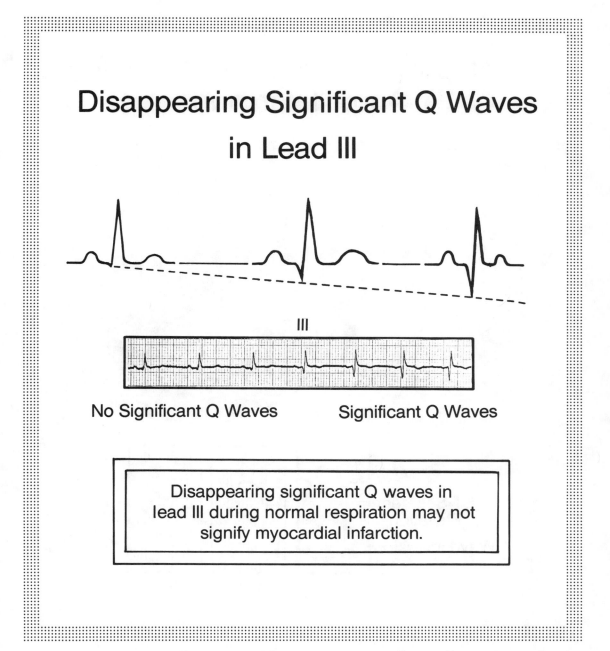

Disappearing Significant Q Waves in Lead III

III

No Significant Q Waves   Significant Q Waves

Disappearing significant Q waves in
lead III during normal respiration may not
signify myocardial infarction.

Not all Q waves signify infarction of the heart, even if they are *significant*. A Q wave in lead III may vary in size with respiration in a normal person because of slight vectorial shifts during respiration. Conversely, this *does not* mean that a Q wave in lead III may not be the result of a myocardial infarction. It is more likely to represent myocardial infarction if it is associated with Q waves in leads II and aVF. Serial electrocardiograms are helpful in providing the answer.

Ventricular Aneurysm Resembling Acute Infarction

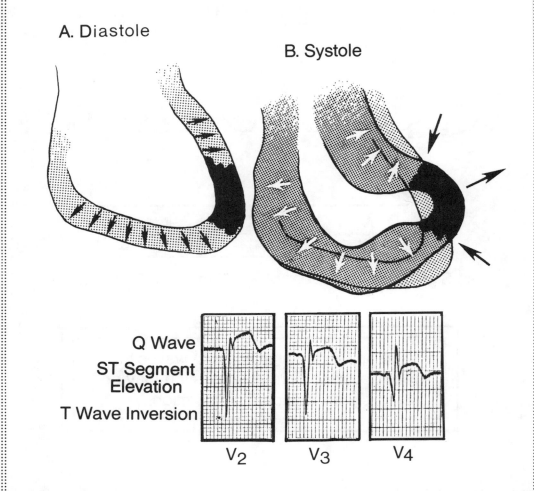

A. Diastole

B. Systole

Q Wave
ST Segment Elevation
T Wave Inversion

V₂   V₃   V₄

This electrocardiogram, with Q waves, elevated ST segments and inverted T waves, could be mistaken for a representation of an acute myocardial infarction. Actually it is from a patient with a *ventricular aneurysm,* following a myocardial infarction that occurred years ago. A ventricular aneurysm is an outpouching (during systole, B above) of a section of scarred ventricular myocardium. In order to exclude an acute myocardial infarction, always ask for comparison electrocardiograms.

Practice
ECG Analysis

Practice
ECG Analysis

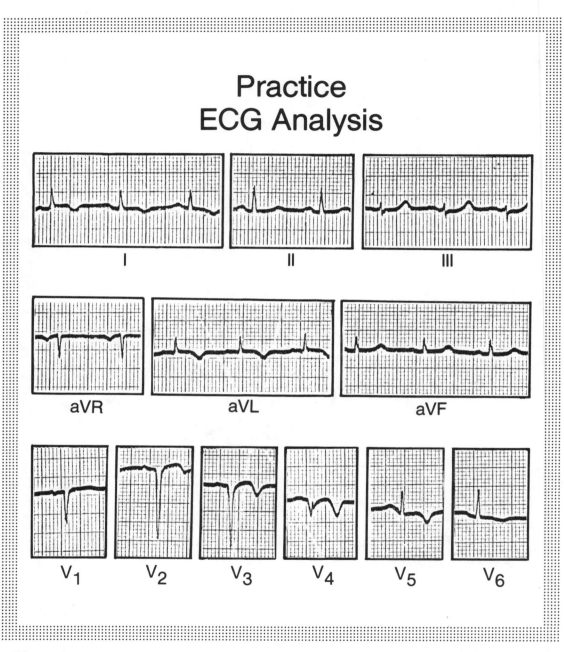

The patient is a 67 year old woman recovering from a heart attack suffered three weeks earlier.

Analysis:

ECG ANALYSIS

1. Rhythm and Rate
   Rhythm: Sinus Rhythm
   Rate: 85/min.
   PR Interval: 0.16 sec.
2. QRS Complex
   Duration: 0.08 sec.
   Axis: $+30°$
   QS complexes, leads V_1 to V_4
3. Ventricular Repolarization
   ST Segment: Elevated in leads V_2 and V_3
   T Wave: Inverted in leads 1, aVL, V_2 to V_6 QRS-T angle wide
4. QT Interval: 0.36 sec.

Impression and Comment

Anterior Myocardial Infarction, Recent
Evolving Ventricular Repolarization (ST-T) Abnormalities

The rounded and/or elevated ST segments seen in leads V_2, V_3 and V_4 followed by the inverted T waves are evolutionary changes following a recent myocardial infarction. The classic electrocardiographic findings in myocardial infarction are seen here.

1. The Q wave = Infarct
2. ST segment elevation = Injury
3. T wave inversion = Ischemia

Practice
ECG Analysis

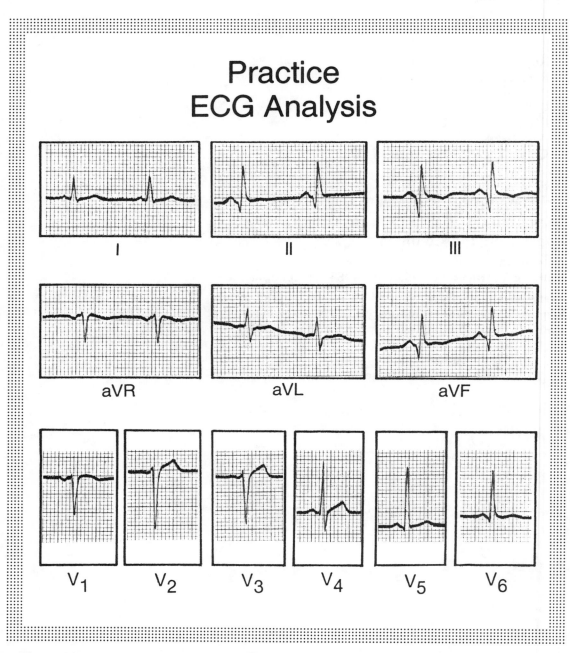

The patient is a 71 year old woman with a history of a heart attack three years earlier. She becomes short of breath on moderate exertion.

Analysis:

ECG ANALYSIS

1. Rhythm and Rate
   Rhythm: Sinus Rhythm
   Rate: 78 / min.
   PR Interval: 0.14 sec.
2. QRS Complex
   Duration: 0.09 sec.
   Axis: +60°
   Significant Q waves, leads II, III and aVF
3. Ventricular Repolarization
   ST Segment: Neither significantly elevated nor depressed
   T Wave: Low, but positive in leads I, aVL, V_5 and V_6
       flat or transitional in lead II
       QRS-T angle wide
4. QT Interval: 0.32 sec.

Impression and Comment

Inferior (Diaphragmatic) myocardial infarction, old
Ventricular Repolarization Abnormalities

This elderly patient, who had a normal electrocardiogram prior to the myocardial infarction, was left with a compromised coronary circulation as a result of the infarct. Evaluation revealed substantial coronary heart disease.

Chapter 5

Conduction Disturbances

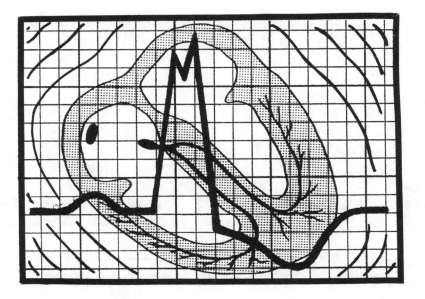

1. Atrioventricular (AV) Conduction Disturbances

2. Intraventricular (IV) Conduction Disturbances

As noted earlier, the heart possesses its own *specialized conduction system.* The impulse originates in the sinoatrial (SA) node and spreads through the atria. The excitation then reaches the atrioventricular (AV) node, located in the right atrium near the tricuspid valve. Conduction proceeds to the bundle of His, then to the left and right bundle branches (LBB and RBB). The impulse then enters the Purkinje system, and ventricular depolarization proceeds from endocardium to epicardium.

Atrioventricular Conduction Disturbances

First Degree AV Block

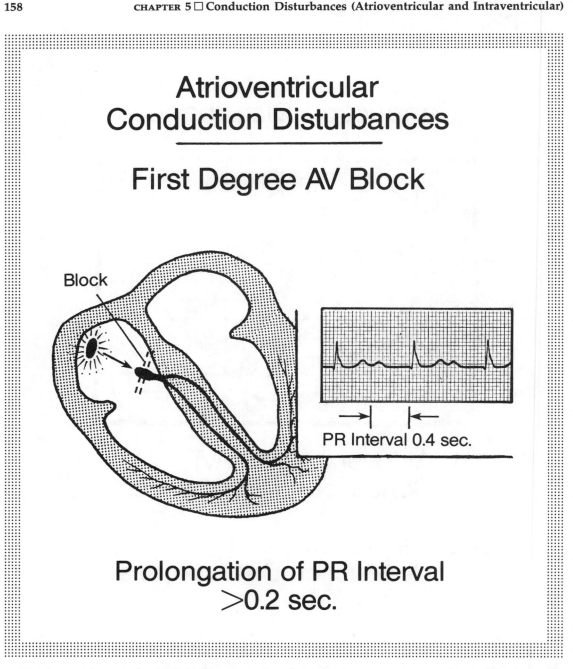

Block

PR Interval 0.4 sec.

Prolongation of PR Interval >0.2 sec.

First degree atrioventricular (AV) block represents a delay in the transmission of impulses from the atria to the ventricles. The delay commonly occurs in the AV node but may occur below the bundle of His. *A prolonged PR interval (greater than 0.2 second)* is seen on this electrocardiogram.

Second Degree AV Block

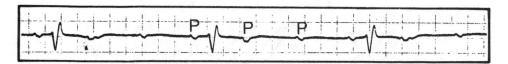

2:1 AV Block

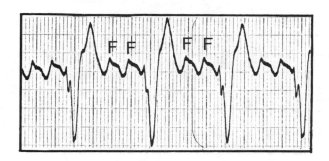

3:1 AV Block

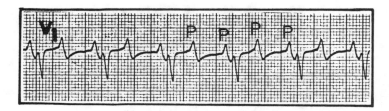

4:1 AV Block

When the ventricles do not respond to atrial stimuli, the P wave is not followed by a QRS complex. The various grades of *second degree AV block* are recognized by the frequency and characteristics of the blocked atrial conduction. In the above electrocardiograms there are two, three and four atrial deflections (P waves, or flutter waves) for every ventricular deflection (QRS complex), respectively.

Second Degree AV Block
(Wenckebach Block)
(Mobitz I Block)

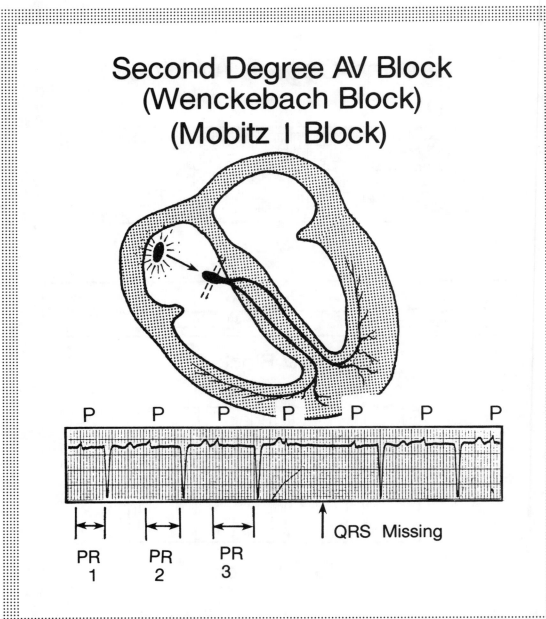

In Mobitz 1 block ventricular beats are "dropped" in a cyclic manner. The PR interval is less prolonged at first but becomes progressively longer, until an atrial contraction no longer initiates a ventricular response. The cycle is then resumed. In the above electrocardiogram, the first PR interval is shorter than the second, which is shorter than the third. The fourth P wave does not conduct and is therefore not followed by a QRS complex. The fifth P wave starts the cycle again.

Second Degree AV Block
(Mobitz II Block)

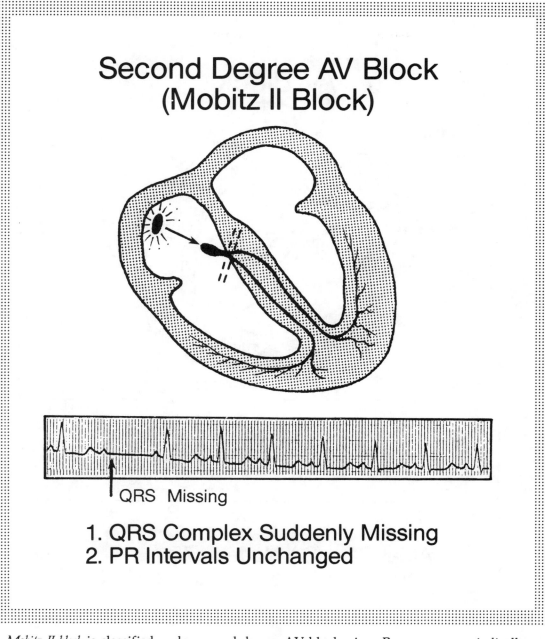

QRS Missing

1. QRS Complex Suddenly Missing
2. PR Intervals Unchanged

Mobitz II block is classified under second degree AV block, since P waves are periodically not followed by QRS complexes (arrow). Electrophysiologic studies have shown that the site of block is usually below the AV node and may be a warning of future complete AV block.

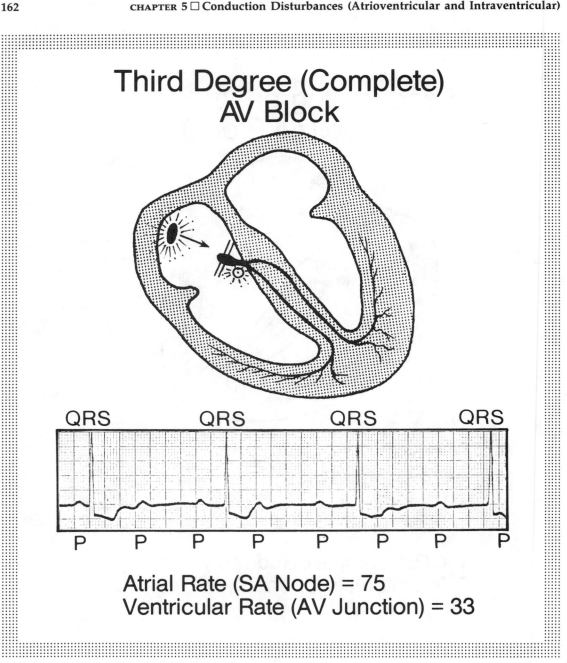

Third Degree (Complete) AV Block

QRS   QRS   QRS   QRS

P   P   P   P   P   P   P   P

Atrial Rate (SA Node) = 75
Ventricular Rate (AV Junction) = 33

In *third degree,* or *complete AV block,* there is no relationship between the atria and the ventricles. The atria, remaining under the control of the SA node, are beating at 75 per minute and are completely dissociated from the ventricles. Depending on the site of impulse formation, the QRS complexes may be of normal duration, as above, with the pacemaker in the AV junction, or quite wide and bizarre, with the pacemaker low in the ventricles. The ventricular rate is 33 per minute.

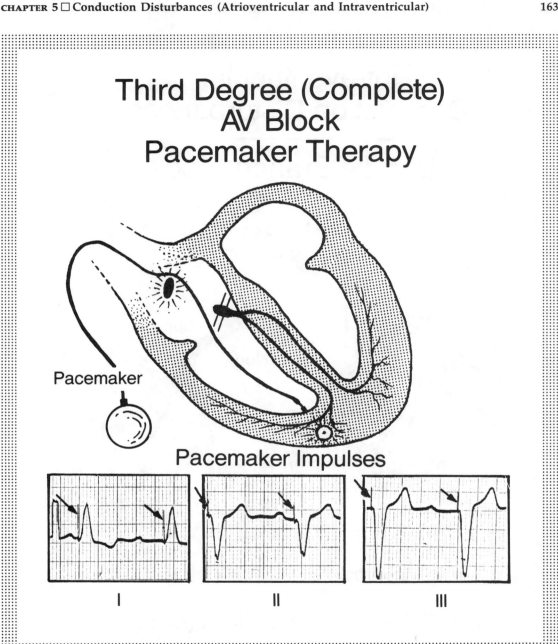

Third Degree (Complete)
AV Block
Pacemaker Therapy

Pacemaker

Pacemaker Impulses

I   II   III

A patient with complete AV block, as seen here, may present with symptoms of cerebral insufficiency, such as dizziness or clouded mentation, or may actually have lost consciousness (Adams-Stokes syndrome) as a result of the low heart rate and poor cardiac output or of transient ventricular standstill or fibrillation. The present-day treatment is electrical pacing to maintain a proper rate and good cardiac output. The arrows point to pacemaker impulses.

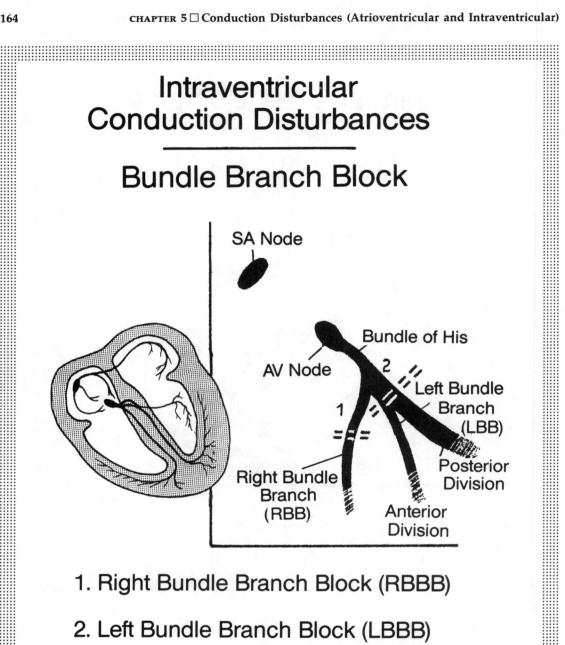

Intraventricular Conduction Disturbances

Bundle Branch Block

1. Right Bundle Branch Block (RBBB)

2. Left Bundle Branch Block (LBBB)

Bundle branch block refers to an interference with conduction in either the right bundle branch or the left bundle branch. The left bundle branch is very short and branches early into an anterior and a posterior division. The right bundle branch, on the other hand, continues almost to the apex of the right ventricle before branching.

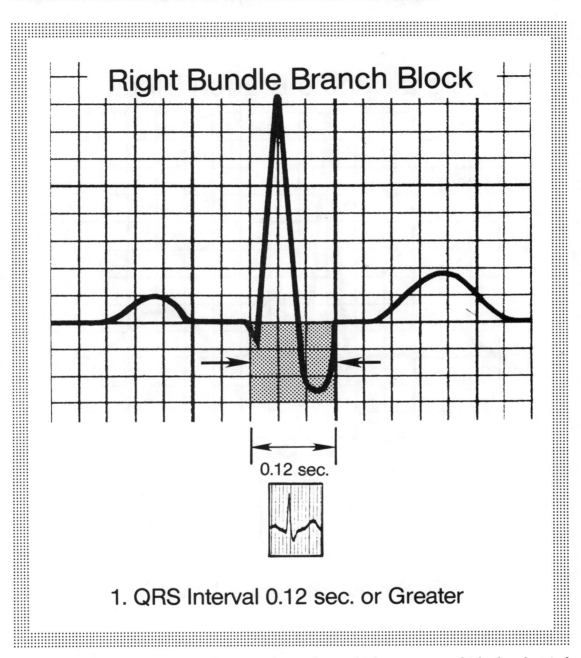

Right Bundle Branch Block

0.12 sec.

1. QRS Interval 0.12 sec. or Greater

The conduction system is similar to a series of superhighways over which the electrical impulse travels. If there is a block in any of these pathways, as above, in *right bundle branch block (RBBB)*, the impulse has to travel through *muscle* tissue, where conduction is delayed. A delay in depolarization therefore, results in a *prolongation of the QRS interval* (QRS complex duration).

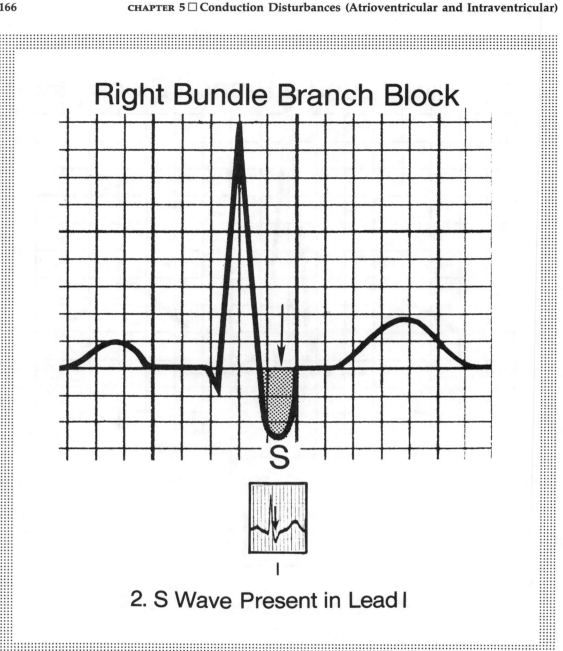

Right Bundle Branch Block

S

I

2. S Wave Present in Lead I

Regardless of where the block may be in right bundle branch block, early depolarization will already have occurred. Only the *terminal* QRS vector is affected by right bundle branch block. This is important, since the electrocardiographic manifestations of initial QRS vector abnormalities, such as the Q waves in myocardial infarction, are not obscured. This *terminal delay* is to the *right,* inscribing the S wave in lead I.

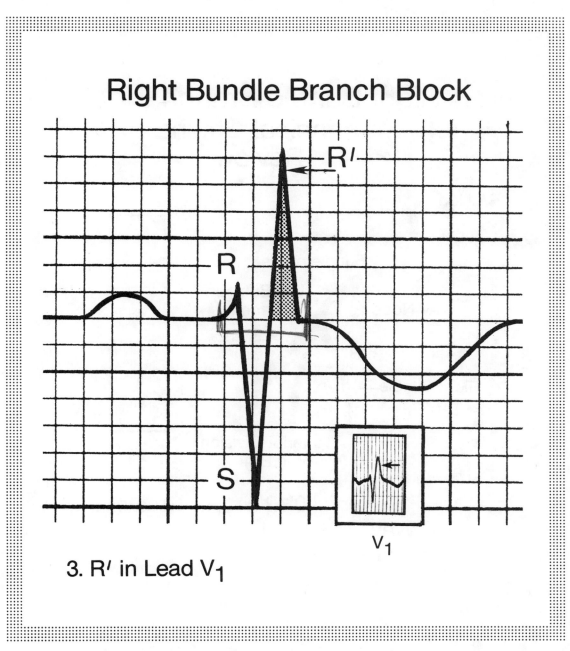

Right Bundle Branch Block

3. R′ in Lead V₁

The *terminal* QRS vector, which is affected by right bundle branch block, is not only to the right, resulting in an *S wave in lead I,* but also *anterior,* producing a second R wave known as an *R′ in lead V₁.* The terminal QRS vector moves toward lead V₁.

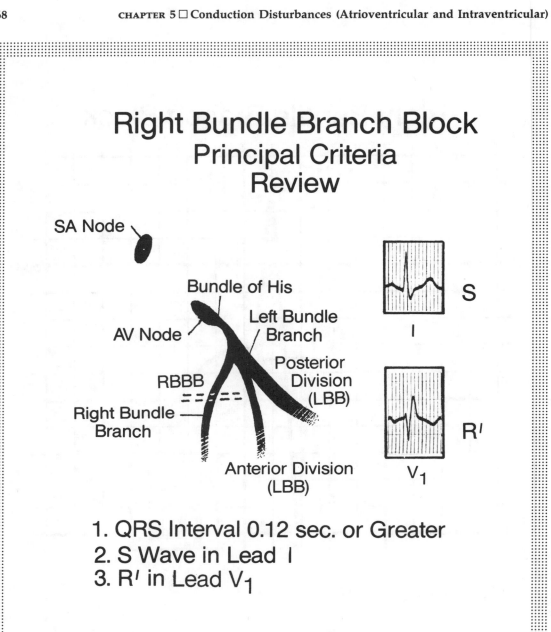

Right Bundle Branch Block
Principal Criteria
Review

1. QRS Interval 0.12 sec. or Greater
2. S Wave in Lead I
3. R' in Lead V_1

   Right bundle branch block is easily recognized by these three characteristics. Right bundle branch block may be found as a congenital condition without any clinical evidence of heart disease. It may also be found in association with an enlarged right ventricle, myocardial infarction and hypertensive cardiovascular disease.

Left Bundle Branch Block

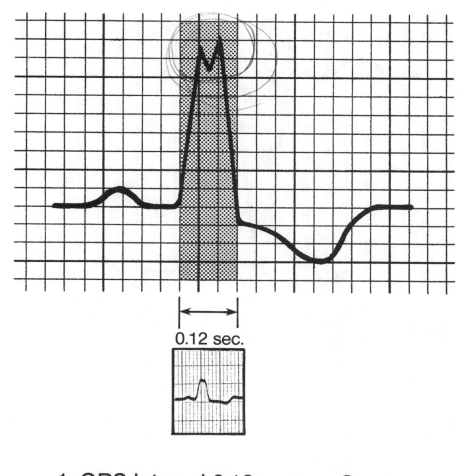

0.12 sec.

1. QRS Interval 0.12 sec. or Greater

In *left bundle branch block (LBBB),* as in right bundle branch block, the QRS complex is prolonged. The delay in conduction is caused by the block, with the electrical impulse having been forced to travel through *muscle* tissue, where conduction is slower.

Left Bundle Branch Block

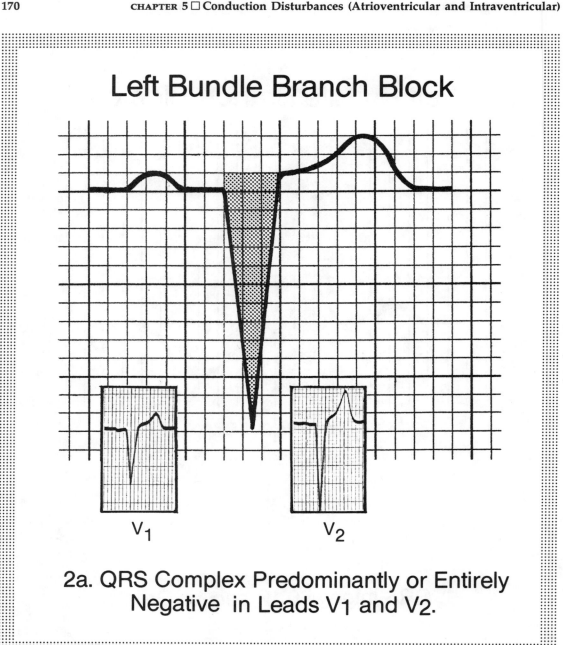

V_1 V_2

2a. QRS Complex Predominantly or Entirely Negative in Leads V_1 and V_2.

In left bundle branch block, in contrast with right bundle branch block, the entire sequence of ventricular depolarization is altered. Both the initial and terminal QRS vectorial forces point more leftward and posteriorly in comparison with the findings in normal conduction. Therefore, the initial R waves seen in the normal electrocardiogram in leads V_1, V_2 and V_3 are much smaller and have often disappeared in leads V_1 and V_2, simulating anterior myocardial infarction. Left ventricular hypertrophy may also be simulated because of the size of the complexes.

Left Bundle Branch Block

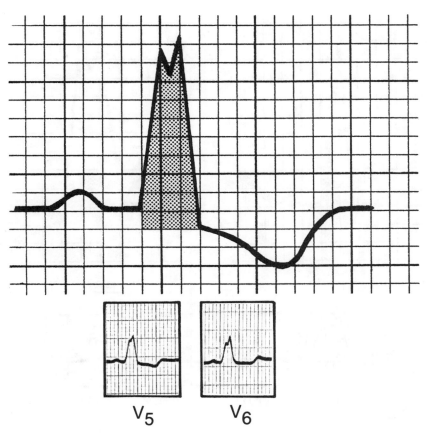

V_5 V_6

2b. QRS Complex Predominantly Positive in Leads V_5 and V_6 and Often Notched

The mean QRS vector, oriented more leftward and posteriorly, which causes leads V_1 and V_2 to be predominantly or entirely *negative,* causes leads V_5 and V_6 to be predominantly or entirely *positive.* The QRS complex in these leads is often notched. Left bundle branch block is often associated with organic disease of the left ventricle.

Left Bundle Branch Block

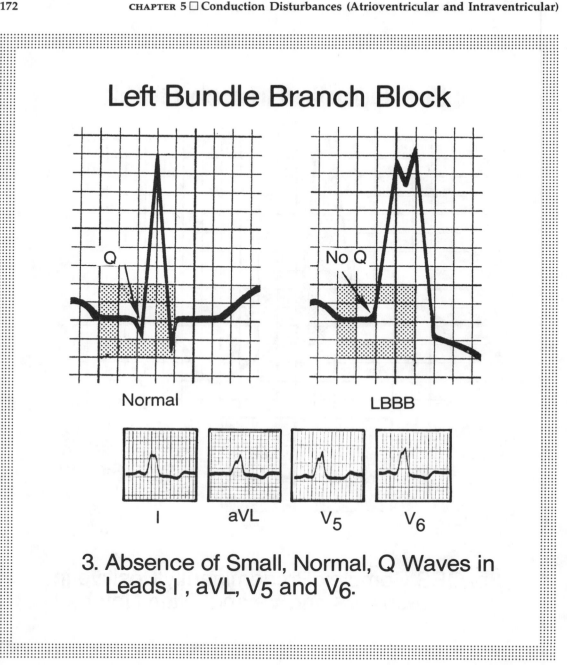

Normal

LBBB

| I | aVL | V$_5$ | V$_6$ |

3. Absence of Small, Normal, Q Waves in Leads I , aVL, V$_5$ and V$_6$.

With the more leftward orientation of the mean QRS vector, the *small* Q waves *normally* seen in leads I, aVL, V$_5$ and V$_6$ disappear. The Q waves of a well-documented myocardial infarction may disappear with the onset of left bundle branch block, masking the electrocardiographic evidence of the infarction.

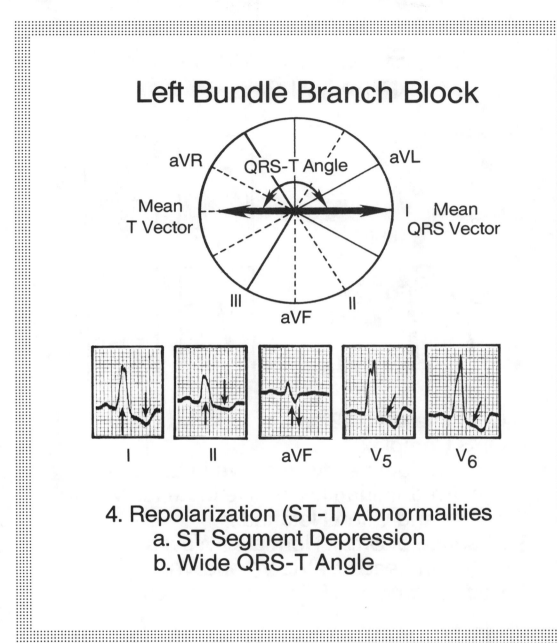

Left Bundle Branch Block

4. Repolarization (ST-T) Abnormalities
a. ST Segment Depression
b. Wide QRS-T Angle

The repolarization alterations occurring with left bundle branch block may be marked. Note that where the QRS complex is positive the T wave is negative, and the transition is shared at lead aVF. The QRS-T angle, is therefore, very wide and the ST segment is depressed.

Left Bundle Branch Block
Principal Criteria
Review

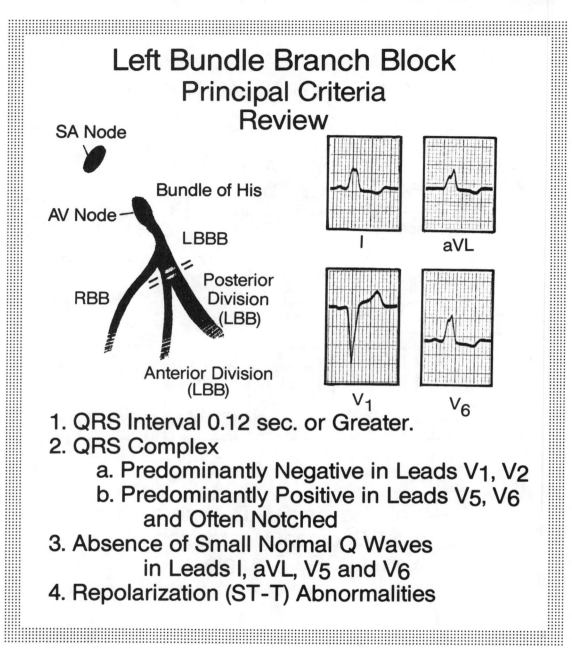

1. QRS Interval 0.12 sec. or Greater.
2. QRS Complex
   a. Predominantly Negative in Leads V_1, V_2
   b. Predominantly Positive in Leads V_5, V_6
      and Often Notched
3. Absence of Small Normal Q Waves
      in Leads I, aVL, V_5 and V_6
4. Repolarization (ST-T) Abnormalities

Do not make the diagnosis of anterior or anteroseptal myocardial infarction from the lack of R waves in the right precordial leads in the presence of left bundle branch block. Also, do not exclude the diagnosis of myocardial infarction in the presence of left bundle branch block. Owing to the size of the complexes, especially leads V_1 and V_2, left ventricular hypertrophy may be simulated by left bundle branch block.

The Hemiblocks

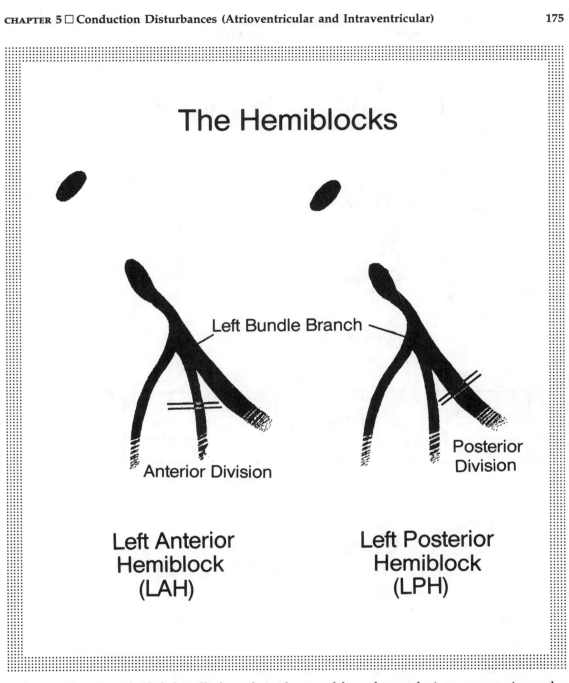

As noted earlier, the left bundle branch is short and branches early into an anterior and a posterior division. The term *hemiblock* refers to a block in either of the two divisions, the anterior *(left anterior hemiblock, LAH)* or the posterior *(left posterior hemiblock, LPH)*.

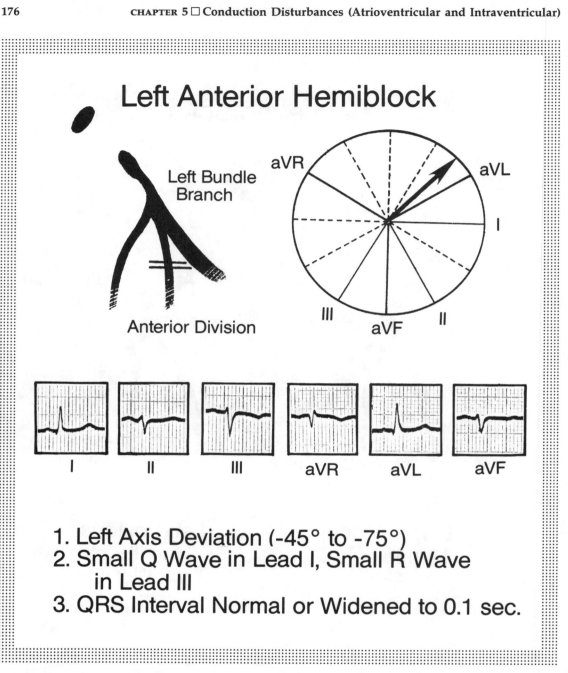

Left Anterior Hemiblock

Left Bundle Branch

Anterior Division

1. Left Axis Deviation (-45° to -75°)
2. Small Q Wave in Lead I, Small R Wave in Lead III
3. QRS Interval Normal or Widened to 0.1 sec.

Left anterior hemiblock, a conduction disturbance in the anterior division of the left bundle branch, is characterized by a marked *left axis deviation* of the mean QRS vector. Note that the QRS complexes in leads II and aVF are predominantly negative, with lead I positive. The QRS complex may be normal or only minimally widened, since a pathway of conduction still remains intact for the electrical impulse to traverse without passage through myocardial tissue.

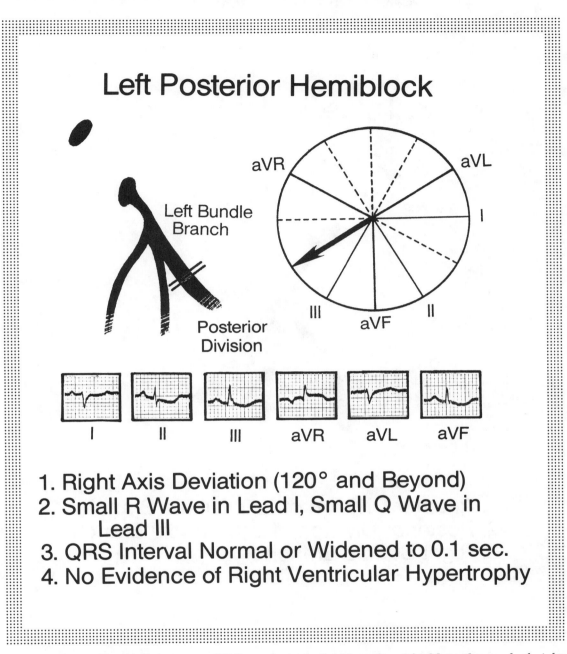

Left Posterior Hemiblock

1. Right Axis Deviation (120° and Beyond)
2. Small R Wave in Lead I, Small Q Wave in Lead III
3. QRS Interval Normal or Widened to 0.1 sec.
4. No Evidence of Right Ventricular Hypertrophy

In *left posterior hemiblock* the mean QRS vector is deviated to the *right*. Note the marked right axis deviation, with the QRS complex almost entirely negative in lead I. There should be no evidence of right ventricular hypertrophy when making the diagnosis of left posterior hemiblock. Right ventricular hypertrophy may also cause marked right axis deviation.

The Trifascicular System

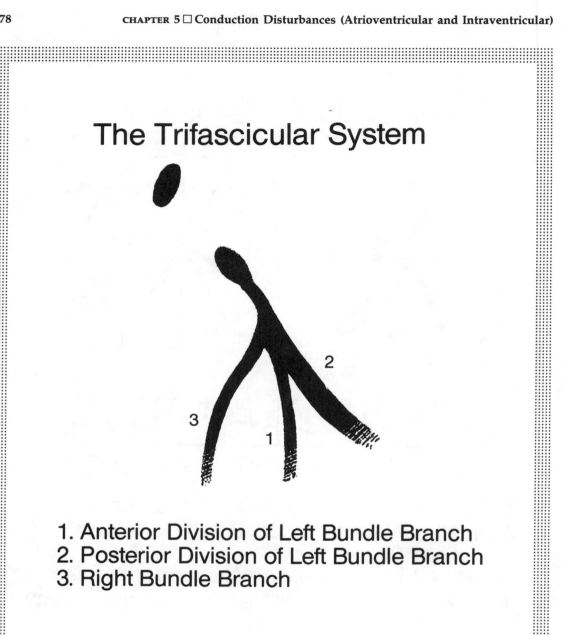

1. Anterior Division of Left Bundle Branch
2. Posterior Division of Left Bundle Branch
3. Right Bundle Branch

Both divisions of the left bundle branch plus the right bundle branch constitute the *trifascicular* system of intraventricular conduction. Each of the three component parts is called a fascicle. Block in two of the three fascicles is commonly seen and is known as bifascicular block.

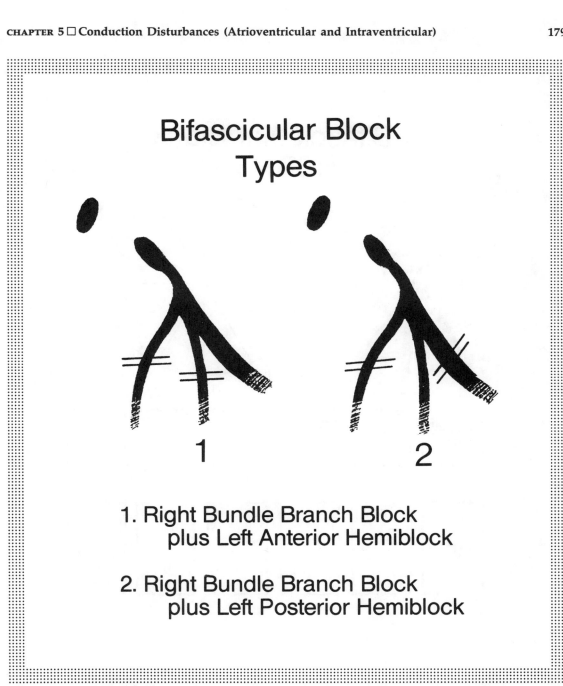

Bifascicular Block Types

1. Right Bundle Branch Block
     plus Left Anterior Hemiblock

2. Right Bundle Branch Block
     plus Left Posterior Hemiblock

Right bundle branch block plus left anterior hemiblock or right bundle branch block plus left posterior hemiblock each involves two of the three fascicles and has been termed *bifascicular* block. Block in all three fascicles would result in complete atrioventricular block.

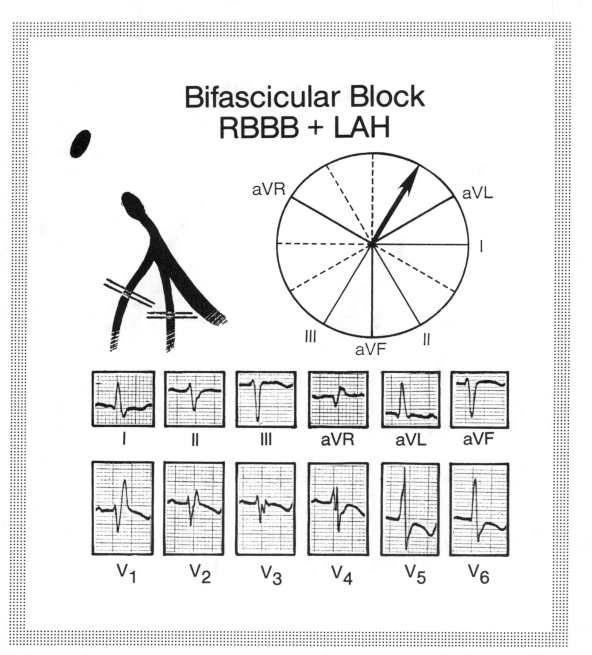

Bifascicular Block
RBBB + LAH

The combination of *right bundle branch block plus left anterior hemiblock (also known as left anterior fascicular block)* is frequently seen. This condition often does not progress to complete atrioventricular block, since the posterior division is a sturdy branch with a dual blood supply. Note the typical right bundle branch block associated with left axis deviation.

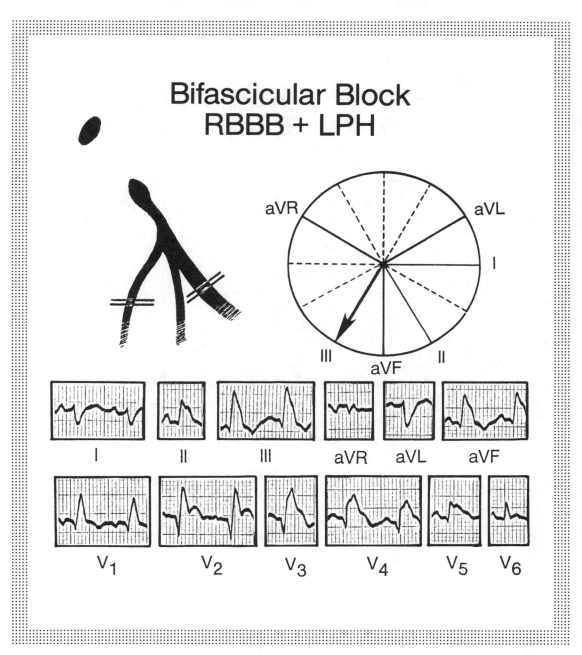

Bifascicular Block
RBBB + LPH

The combination of *right bundle branch block plus left posterior hemiblock (left posterior fascicular block)* may augur ill for the patient, since in this disorder the entire atrioventricular conduction system is dependent on the weakest fascicle, the anterior division, with a single blood supply. These patients must be followed closely; pacemaker therapy must be considered with progress of the disease to the third fascicle. This patient also had an anterior myocardial infarction; hence the initial Q waves in the precordial leads.

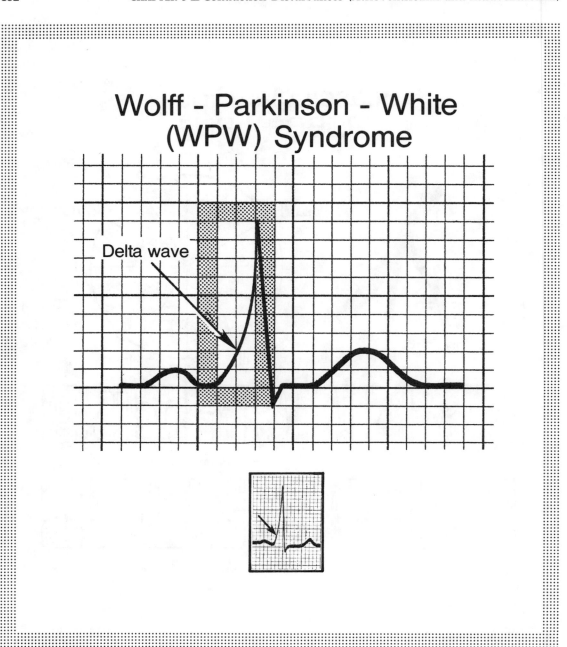

Wolff - Parkinson - White (WPW) Syndrome

Delta wave

The *Wolff-Parkinson-White (WPW) syndrome* represents an anomalous pathway or bypass from the atria to the ventricles. These patients may be subject to attacks of paroxysmal tachycardia. The electrocardiographic characteristics include.

1. Short PR internal (0.12 sec. or less).
2. Prolonged QRS interval (greater than 0.1 sec.).
3. Slurring of the upstroke by a *delta* wave.

Practice
ECG Analysis

Practice
ECG Analysis

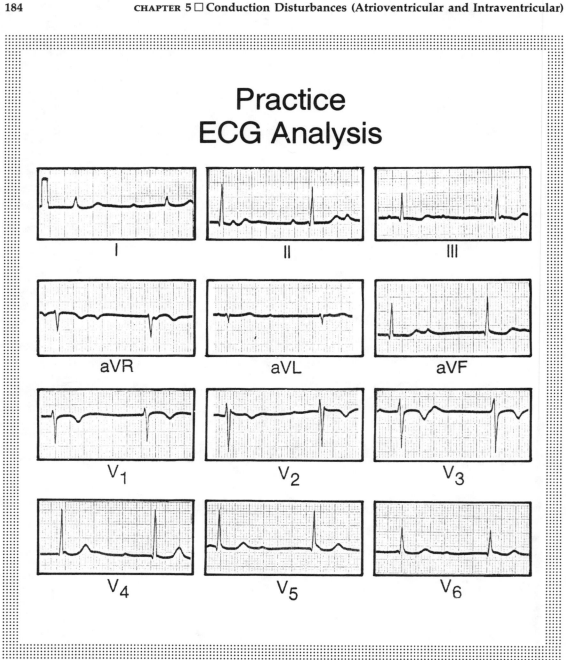

The patient is a 17 year old asymptomatic high school athlete, who was referred because of a low heart rate.

Analysis:

ECG ANALYSIS

1. Rhythm and Rate
   Rhythm: Third Degree (Complete) AV Block
   Rate: Atrial 80/min.
          Ventricular 47/min.
   The atria and ventricles are beating at their own intrinsic rate.
2. QRS Complex
   Duration: 0.08 sec.
   Axis: + 70°
3. Ventricular Repolarization
   ST Segment: neither significantly elevated nor depressed
   T Wave: QRS-T angle normal
4. QT Interval: 0.36 sec.

Impression and Comment

Third Degree (Complete) AV Block, Congenital

The atrial impulses originate in the SA node but do not proceed to the ventricles because of the complete AV block. The QRS complexes are normally narrow, with the AV junction controlling the ventricles. A review of this patient's history and electrocardiograms since birth revealed that he was born with complete AV block. It was decided to permit him to continue all activities with no restrictions except for competitive sports. In the future he may require appropriate therapy, but, to date, he has remained asymptomatic for many years of follow-up, without therapy. This is very different from the patient who develops permanent complete AV block from disease or after heart surgery, which requires immediate pacemaker therapy.

Practice
ECG Analysis

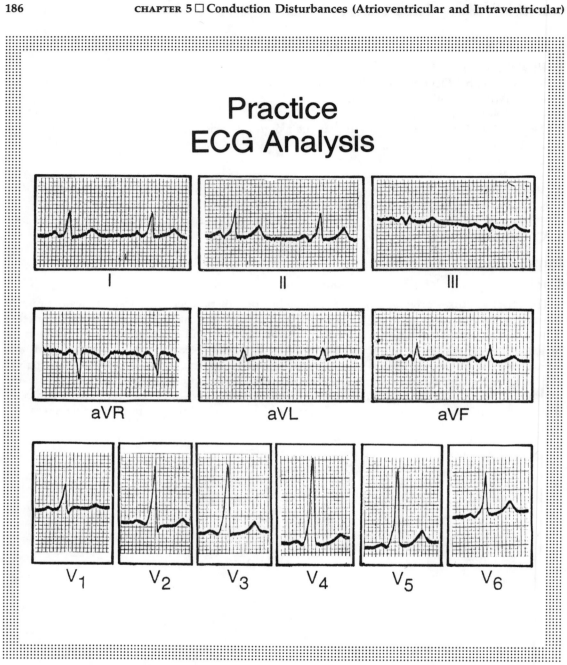

The patient is a 60 year old man with a long history of multiple episodes of heart rhythm disturbances, with a rapid heart rate and recent onset of chest pain during these episodes.

Analysis:

ECG ANALYSIS

1. Rhythm and Rate
   Rhythm: Sinus Rhythm
   Rate: 70/min.
   PR Interval: 0.12 sec.
2. QRS Complex
   Duration: 0.12 sec.
   Axis: + 30°
   The QRS complex has a slurred upstroke (delta wave).
3. Ventricular Repolarization
   ST Segment: neither abnormally elevated nor depressed
   T Wave: Normal QRS-T angle
4. QT Interval: 0.35 sec. (measured from end of delta wave, in lead aVF).

Impression and Comment

Wolff-Parkinson-White (WPW) Syndrome

The short PR interval may be more apparent than real; since the measurement from the beginning of the P wave to the end of the QRS complex may be normal.

There is a frequent association of the WPW syndrome with paroxysmal supraventricular tachycardia. A typical case history is that of an older patient who has had bouts of rapid heart action throughout his life, but who has had chest pain during these episodes only in recent years, owing to increasing age and coronary disease.

Practice
ECG Analysis

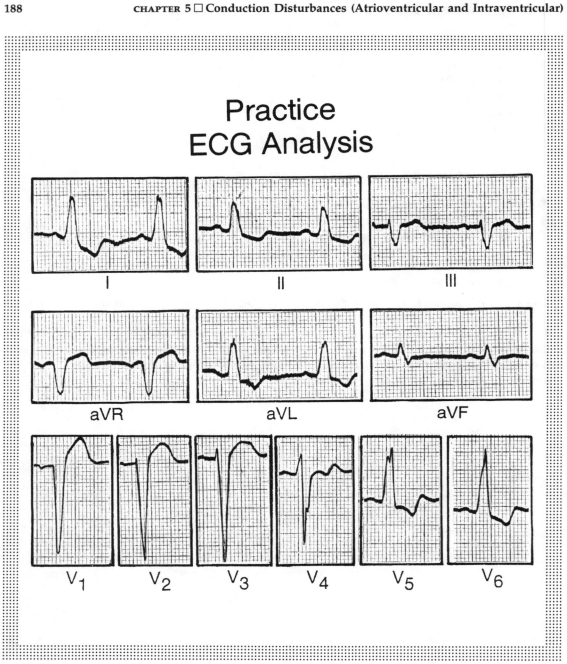

The patient is a 70 year old woman with congestive heart failure. Her medication includes digitalis and diuretics.

Analysis:

ECG ANALYSIS

1. Rhythm and Rate
   Rhythm: Sinus Rhythm
   Rate: 65/min.
   PR Interval: 0.16 sec.
2. QRS Complex
   Duration: 0.14 sec.
   Axis: 0° with a markedly posterior orientation.
   QS complex in lead V_1
   Absence of small normal Q waves in leads I, aVL, V_5 and V_6.
3. Ventricular Repolarization
   ST Segment: Depressed in leads I, II, aVL, V_5 and V_6
   T Wave: Wide QRS-T angle
4. QT Interval: 0.35 sec.

Impression and Comment

Left Bundle Branch Block

This patient also had an old inferior (diaphragmatic) myocardial infarction, completely obscured by the development of the left bundle branch block. Left bundle branch block may simulate myocardial infarction electrocardiographically when none has occurred and may mask myocardial infarction in the presence of clear evidence of its occurrence. This patient also had a large left ventricle, which cannot be determined with certainty in the presence of left bundle branch block.

Chapter 6

Arrhythmias

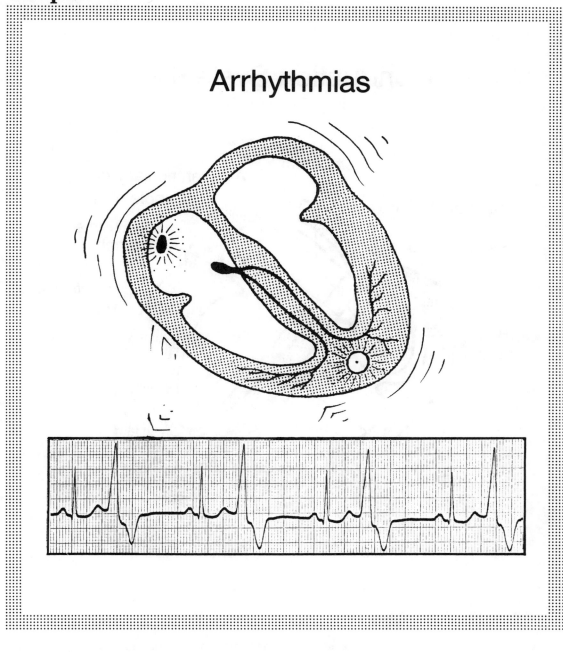

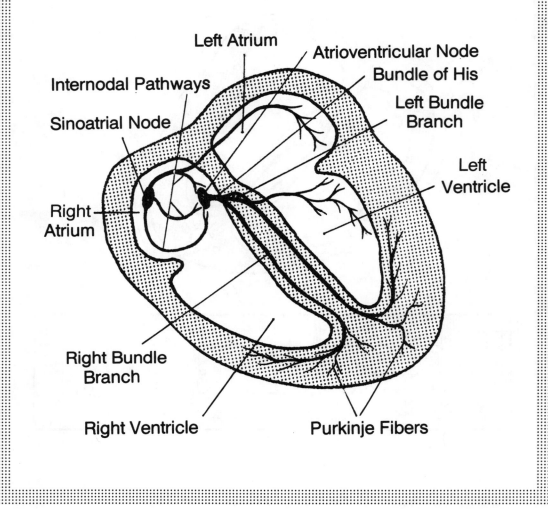

Conduction System of the Heart

The atrioventricular (AV) conduction system of the heart had been discussed earlier. Normally, the sinoatrial (SA) node is the dominant pacemaker of the heart. If it fails, a lower pacemaker may take over. If that one fails, a still lower pacemaker may take over, and so on. Although the dominant pacemaker of the heart is the SA node, under various circumstances and stimuli any part of the specialized conduction system or myocardial tissue may become the dominant pacemaker. There may be two or more pacemakers propagating impulses at the same time. The SA node emits from 60 to 100 impulses per minute, the AV junction from 40 to 60 impulses per minute and still lower pacemakers, such as an idioventricular pacemaker, less than 40 impulses per minute.

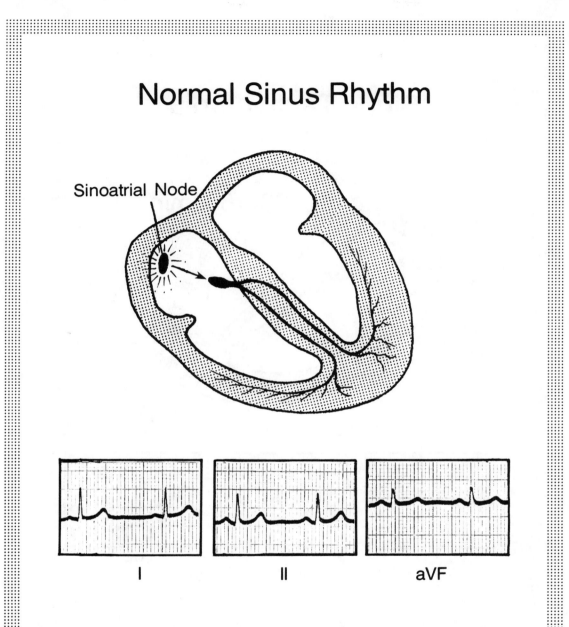

Normal Sinus Rhythm

Sinoatrial Node

I   II   aVF

Before examining rhythm disturbances, let us review the criteria for *normal sinus rhythm*.

1. The mean P vector is normal (the P waves are constant and upright in leads I, II and aVF).
2. Each P wave is followed by a QRS complex, and each QRS complex is preceded by a P wave.
3. The PR interval is from 0.12 to 0.20 sec. (three to five small boxes wide) and constant from beat to beat.
4. The rate is regular, between 60 and 100 beats per minute.

When the word "nodal" is used it refers to the *AV* node and *not* to the SA node. Any beat or rhythm originating outside the *SA node* is an *ectopic* beat or rhythm, ectopic in that it does not originate in the normal site.

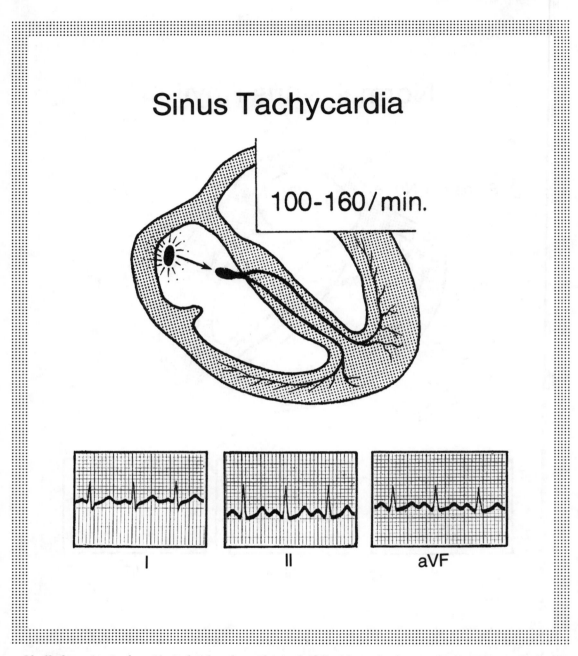

Sinus Tachycardia

100-160/min.

| I | II | aVF |

If all the criteria for sinus rhythm have been fulfilled but the heart rate is greater than 100 beats per minute, the rhythm is called *sinus tachycardia*. Tachycardia means fast heart. The range for sinus tachycardia is 100 to 160 beats per minute.

Sinus Bradycardia

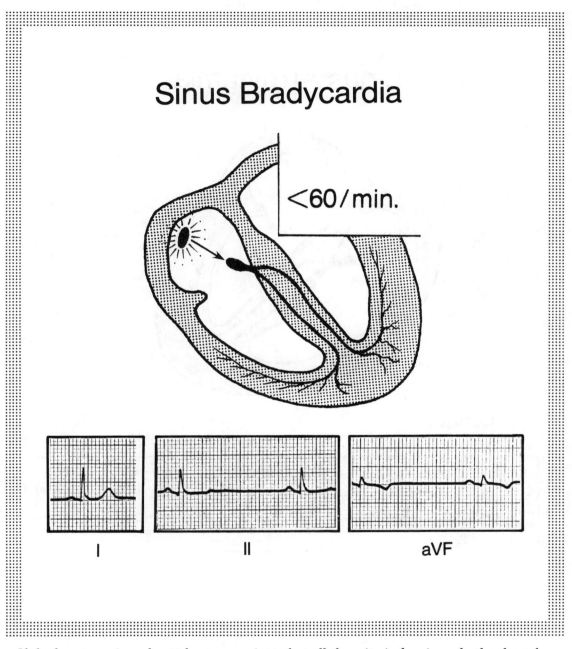

If the heart rate is under 60 beats per minute but all the criteria for sinus rhythm have been fulfilled, the rhythm is known as *sinus bradycardia.* Bradycardia means slow heart.

Sinus Arrhythmia

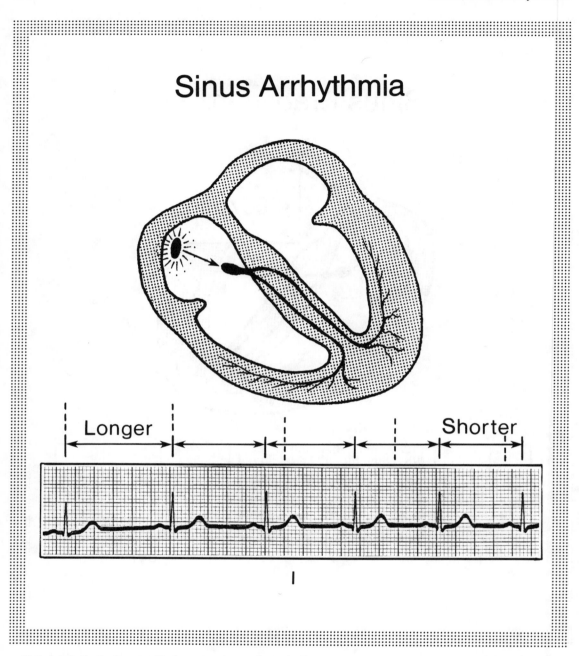

Sinus arrhythmia meets all the criteria as described under normal sinus rhythm, except for the variation in rate, often associated with the respiratory cycles. It is commonly seen in the young. The PR intervals are constant, but the RR intervals are continually changing.

Sinoatrial (SA) Block

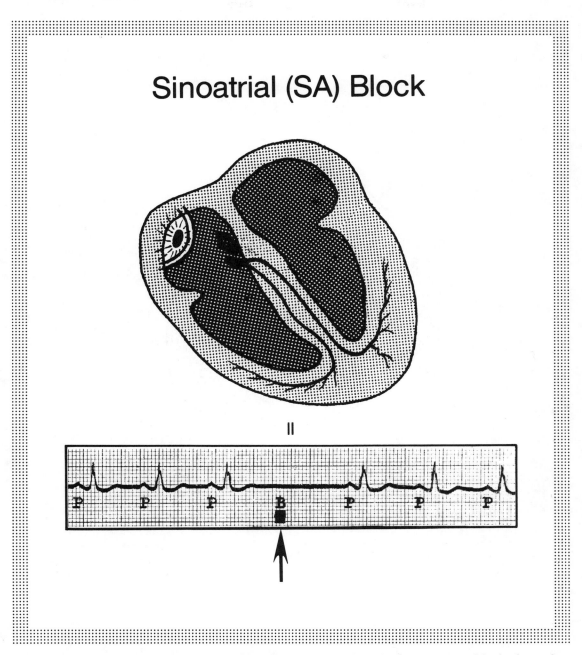

In *sinoatrial (SA) block* the SA node initiates an impulse but the *propagation* is blocked, so that the atria are not depolarized and hence there is no P wave. The pause is a multiple of the regular cycle length. The block, represented by the letter B above, is seen where the P should normally be.

Sinus Arrest

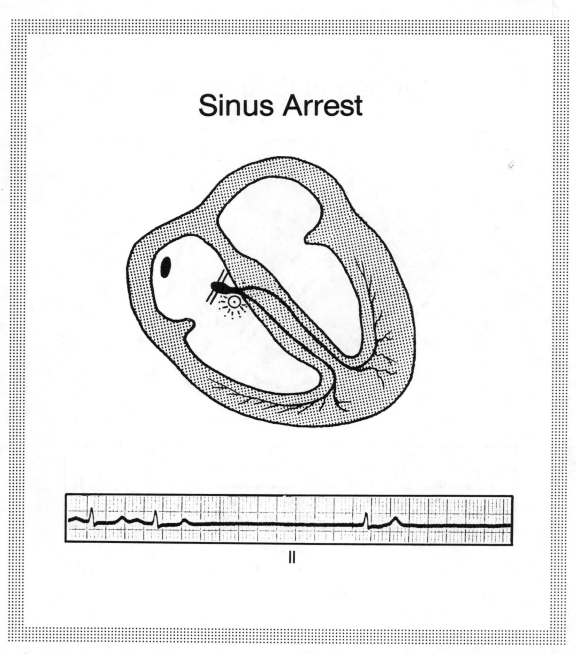

II

Sinus arrest is a sudden failure of the SA node to initiate an expected impulse; it is a failure of impulse *formation* rather than of impulse *propagation*. Fortunately, a lower pacemaker often becomes dominant, initiating a new rhythm (in this case AV junctional—to be described shortly).

Premature Atrial Contraction (PAC)

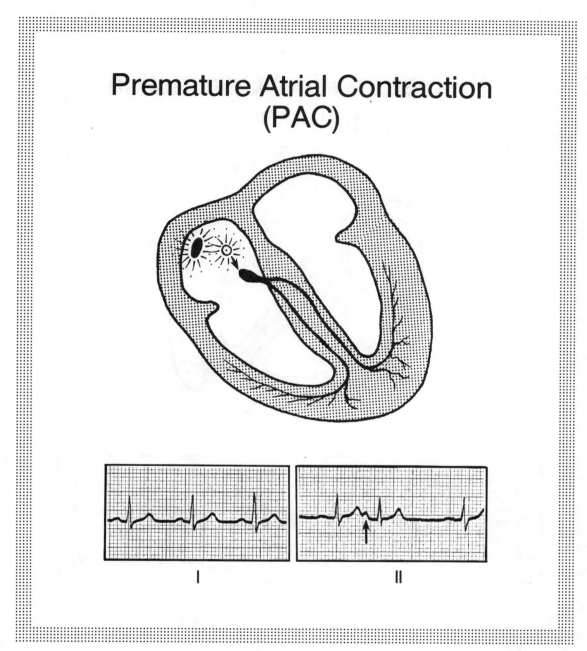

I   II

Premature beats of the atria are seen when an ectopic atrial pacemaker propagates an impulse before the next normal beat is due. The premature beat may be conducted to the ventricles, as seen in lead II. The P wave of the premature beat differs from the sinus P wave in contour. In general, following atrial premature beats, the PR interval may be normal or prolonged, and the QRS complex may be of normal contour and duration or of changed configuration and prolonged, depending on the state of refractoriness of the conduction tissue. Also, the premature beats of the atria may herald paroxysms of atrial tachycardia.

Premature Atrial Contraction
(Blocked)

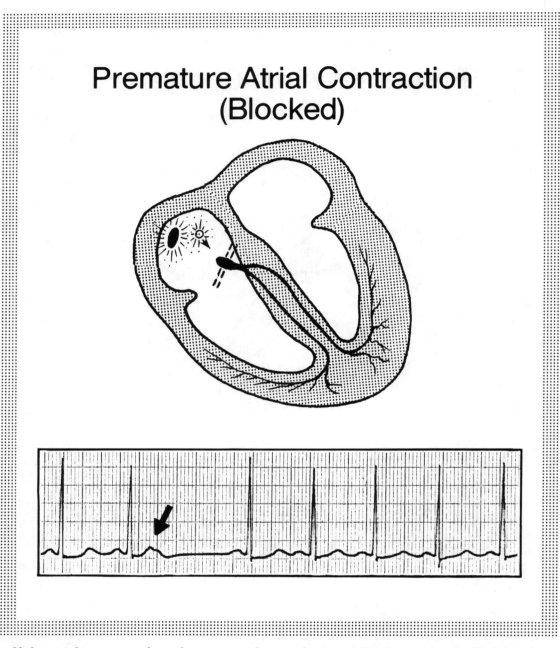

If the atrial premature beat does not conduct to the ventricles, it is said to be *blocked* and not followed by a QRS complex. The arrow points to the *blocked atrial premature beat.* Conduction to the ventricle did not occur because the atria depolarized during the absolute refractory period of the ventricle.

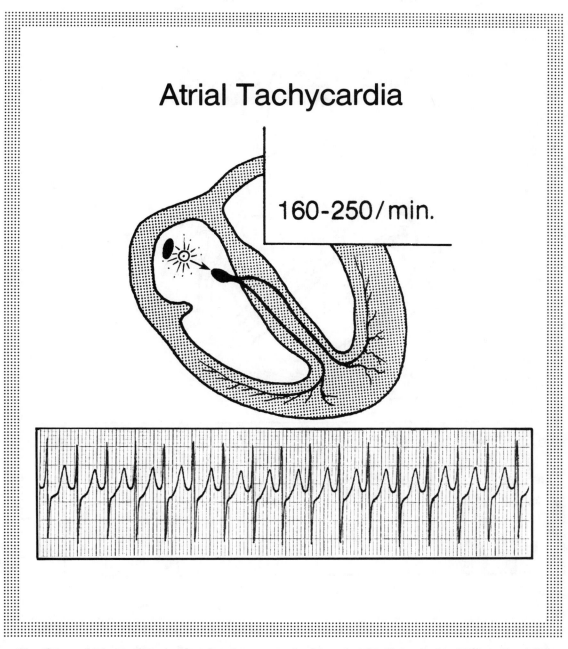

Atrial Tachycardia

160-250/min.

The SA node is no longer the dominant pacemaker. *Atrial tachycardia* is characterized by a rapid (160 to 250 beats per minute) rate and regular rhythm, sudden in onset, often terminating abruptly; it may be followed by a pause. The P waves, when seen, differ from the sinus P waves in contour.

Atrial Tachycardia
2:1 AV Block

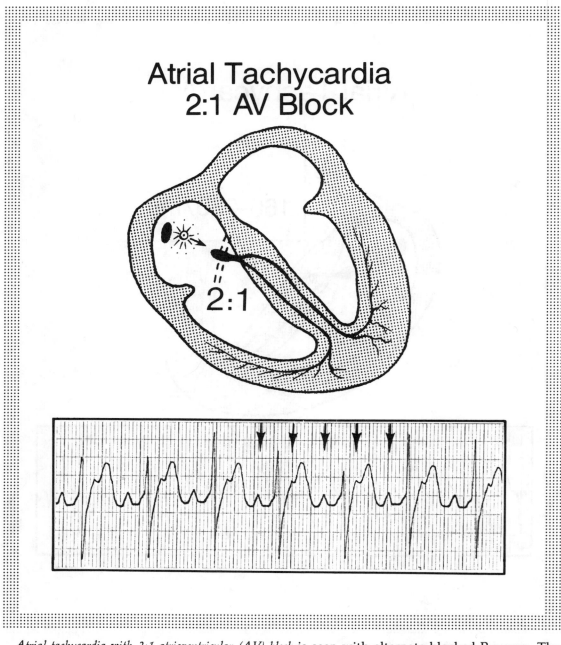

Atrial tachycardia with 2:1 atrioventricular (AV) block is seen with alternate blocked P waves. The arrows on the electrocardiogram point to the P waves. The rhythm is atrial tachycardia because the atria are beating at a rate of 170 per minute. Review second degree AV block, page 159.

Atrial Flutter

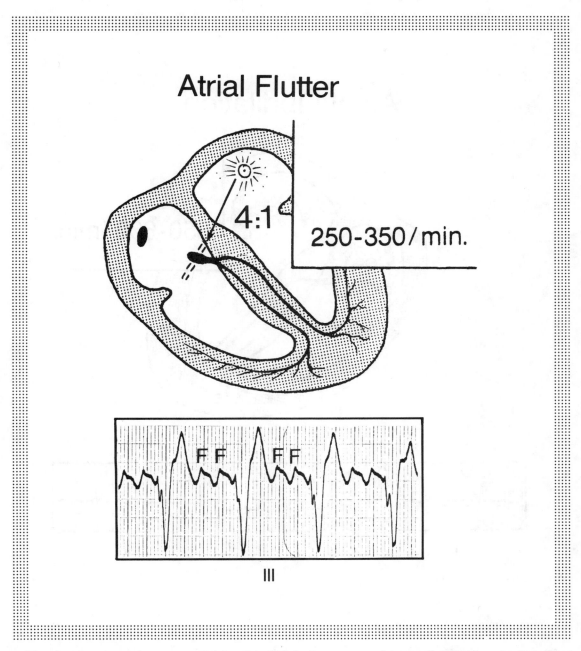

The *fluttering atria* are represented by the undulating waves, rising and falling to the baseline. Note the "saw-tooth" character of the atrial waves (F or flutter waves). The atrial rate is 300 beats per minute, whereas the ventricular rate is 75 beats per minute, with a ratio of 4:1. The atrial rate in atrial flutter is usually 250 to 350 beats per minute. The wide QRS complex is due to this patients left bundle branch block.

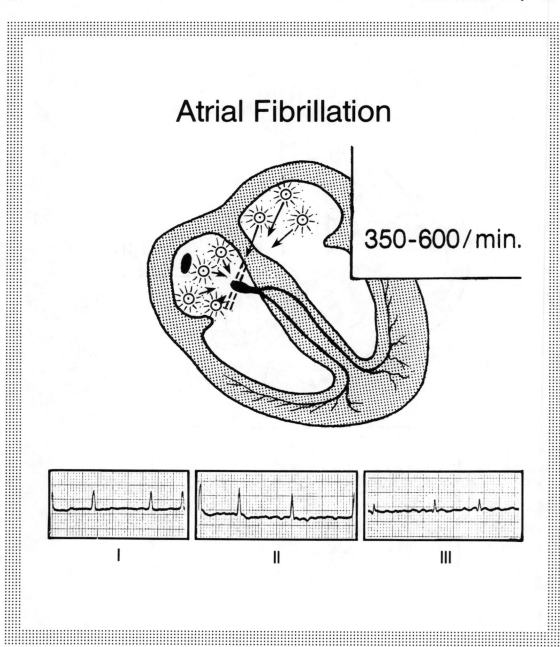

Atrial Fibrillation

350-600/min.

I   II   III

Disorganized, ineffective contractions of the atria (350 to 600 per minute) characterize *atrial fibrillation*. No P waves are seen, and the ventricular response is irregular, depending on how many of the 350 to 600 impulses are conducted to the ventricles. If the atrial rate is 500 per minute and the ventricular rate is 125 per minute, it means that one in four atrial impulses is conducted, irregularly, to the ventricles. This rhythm has been described as irregularly irregular.

Multifocal Atrial Tachycardia

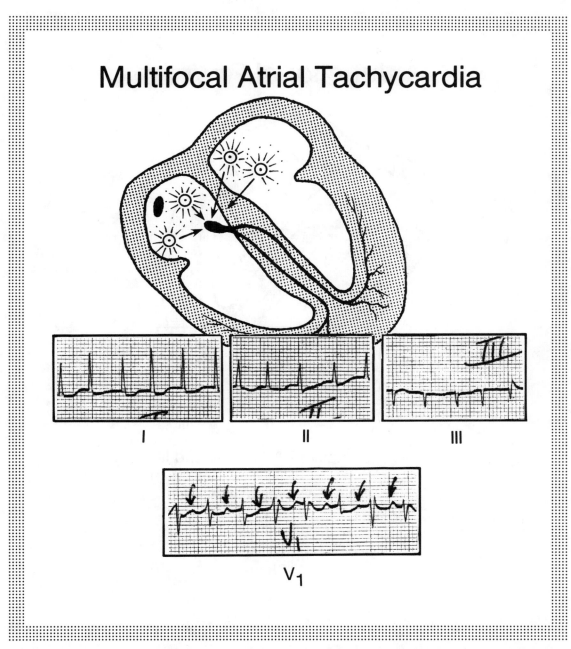

Multifocal (chaotic) atrial tachycardia is sometimes mistaken for atrial filbrillation, since the rhythm is irregularly irregular. At a quick glance, leads I, II and III might appear to be examples of atrial fibrillation. Lead V_1, however, reveals the different P wave contours as well as the varying PR intervals. This rhythm is frequently found in patients with chronic obstructive pulmonary disease associated with hypoxia.

Junctional Rhythm

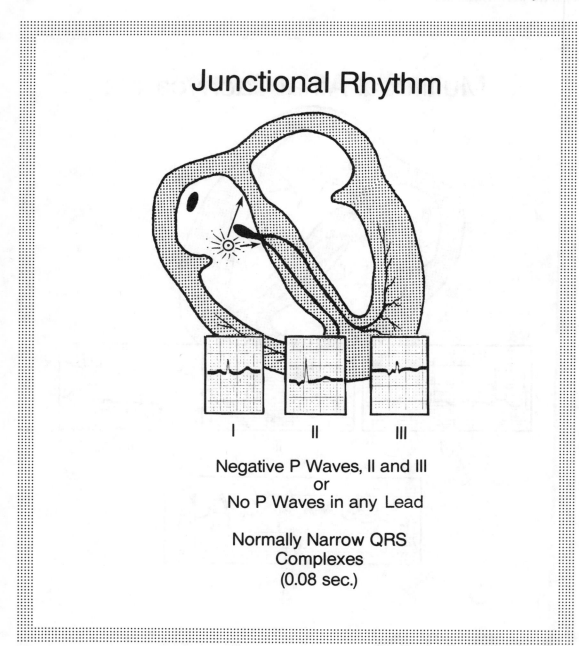

I   II   III

Negative P Waves, II and III
or
No P Waves in any Lead

Normally Narrow QRS
Complexes
(0.08 sec.)

The *atrioventricular (AV) junction* is a lower center of excitation and may become the dominant pacemaker when the SA node is depressed. The AV junctional rate is 40 to 60 beats per minute. The P waves are usually upright in lead I and inverted in leads II and III; they may come before, during or after the QRS complex. If the atria are not depolarized, no P wave will be present. The QRS complexes are generally normal, since ventricular depolarization proceeds normally. When the P wave precedes the QRS complex, as above, the PR interval is usually short, up to 0.12 sec.

Junctional Tachycardia

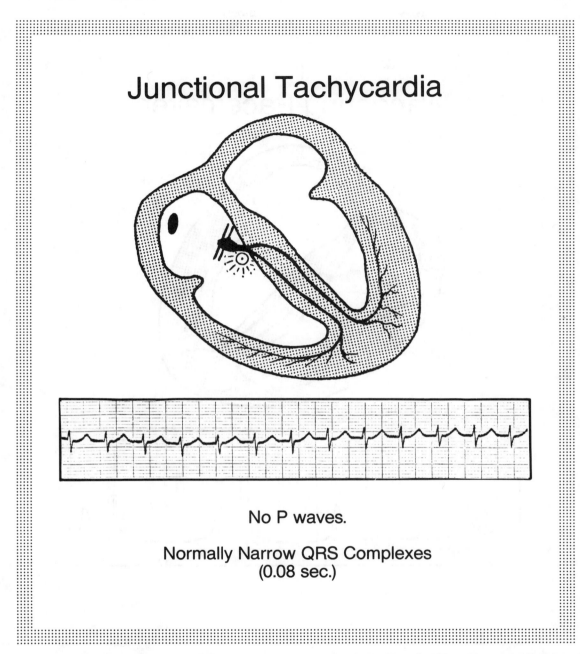

No P waves.

Normally Narrow QRS Complexes
(0.08 sec.)

A junctional rhythm may have negative P waves in leads II, III and aVF and positive P waves in lead I, or no P waves at all. This occurs when the AV junction produces an impulse that proceeds to normally depolarize the ventricles while not depolarizing the atria (illustrated diagrammatically above). At times a tachycardia, as above, is classified under the overall category of *supraventricular tachycardia,* originating above the ventricles.

Wandering Pacemaker

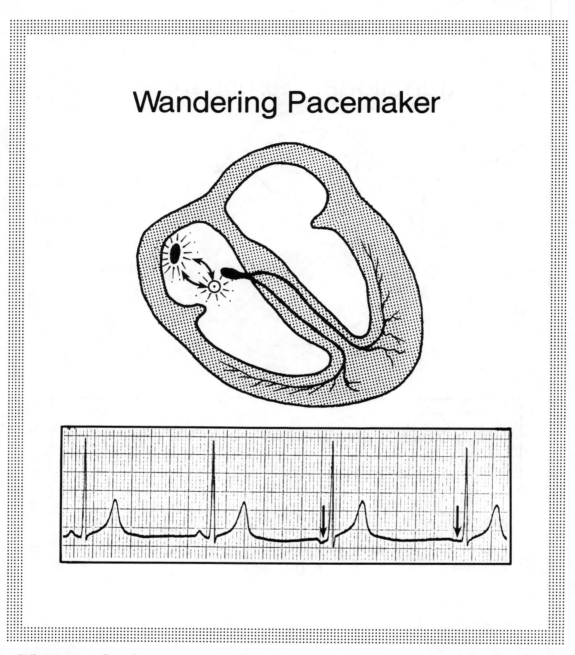

When pacemaker dominance is shared by more than one pacemaker, P waves of varying configurations result. This is known as a *wandering pacemaker.* Here pacemaker dominance is shared by the SA node and a lower pacemaker. Notice the variation in P wave polarity. The arrows point to P waves of different configurations.

Junctional Escape Rhythm with Sinus Arrest

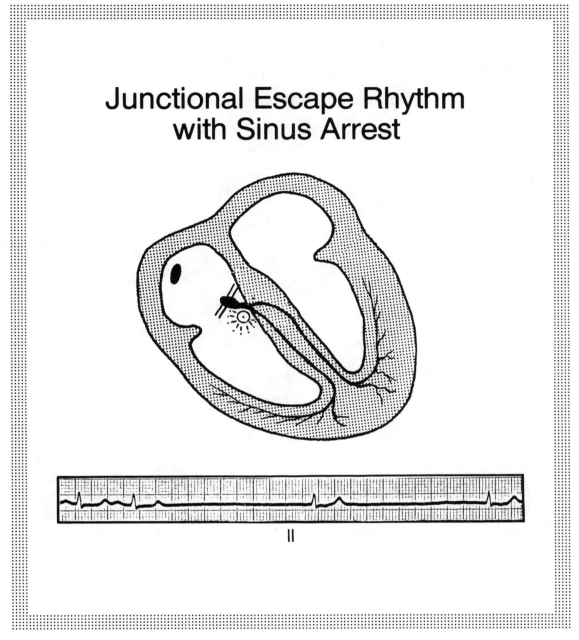

II

With the *arrest of the SA node,* a long pause follows. The beat following this pause is known as an *escape* beat, usually from a lower pacemaker, as shown above. If the pacemaker originating the escape beat remains the dominant one, the rhythm may then be called an *escape rhythm.* In this case the AV junction became the dominant pacemaker.

Premature Ventricular Contractions (PVC)

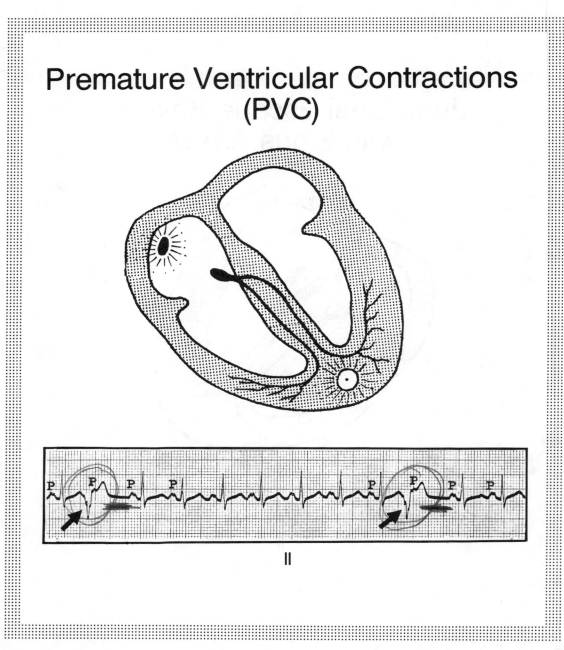

Premature ventricular contractions (PVC, arrows above) are seen when an impulse is propagated from a ventricular focus before the next normal beat is due. The QRS complex is commonly widened and not preceded by a P wave. A longer than usual *(compensatory)* pause follows. There may be retrograde activation of the atria following a premature contraction, or the normal sinus P waves may continue, as above. The sinus P waves following the PVC are blocked because of conduction system refractoriness.

Premature Ventricular Contractions
Bigeminy

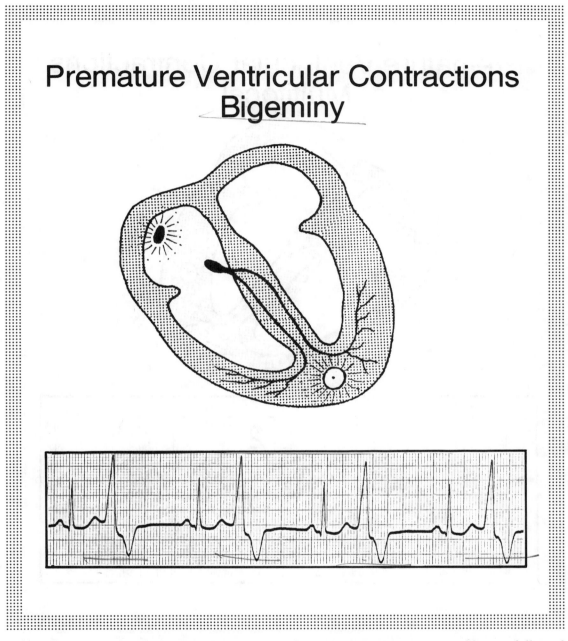

Bigeminy describes the heart beating in groups of two. In this patient, a normal beat is followed by a premature ventricular contraction and is separated from the next group by a pause. Trigeminy refers to heartbeats in groups of three. The words bigeminy and trigeminy do not reveal the components of the group; these must be described.

Premature Ventricular Contractions
Multifocal

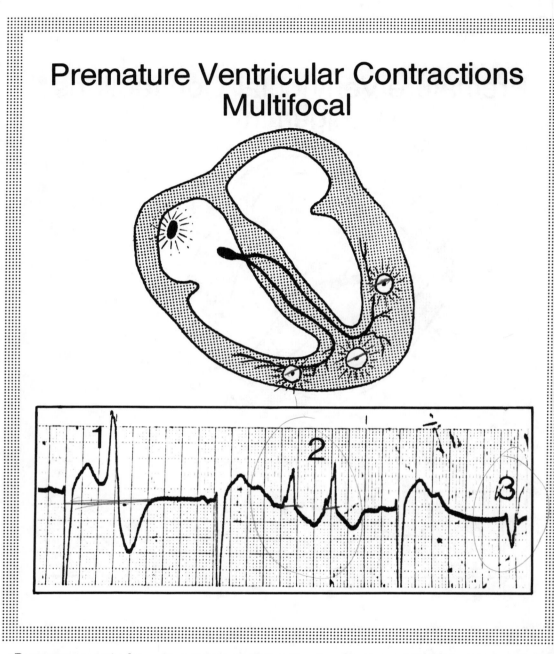

Premature ventricular contractions may be unifocal, as seen on the two previous pages, or multifocal. Above we see premature ventricular contractions from three different foci. This situation may be encountered following myocardial infarction or digitalis toxicity and requires careful attention.

Ventricular Tachycardia

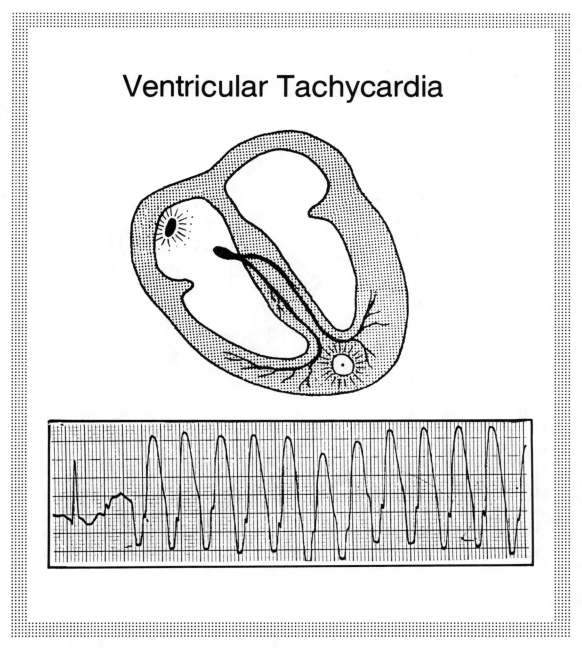

In *ventricular tachycardia* the ectopic pacemaker in the ventricle may produce "runs" of premature ventricular contractions. Once started, ventricular tachycardia may be sustained until terminated spontaneously, by medication or by electrical cardioversion, or it may be intermittent. The QRS complexes are widened and bizarre and the rate is usually from 150 to 250 beats per minute. The rhythm may be regular or slightly irregular. Atrial activity is usually not affected.

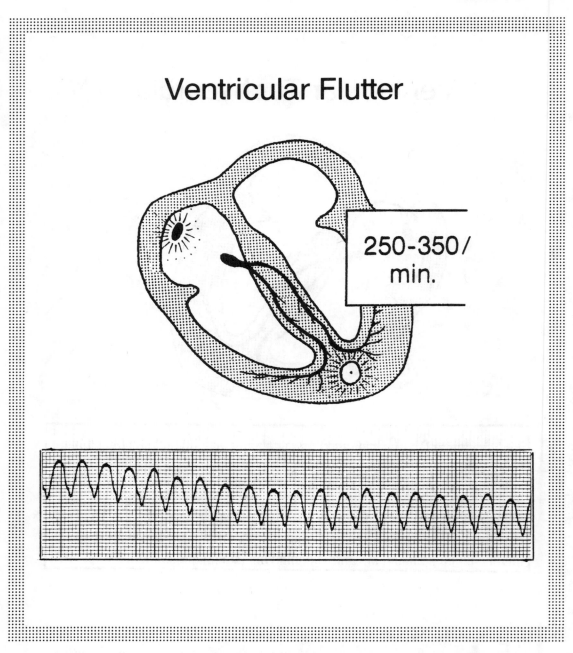

Ventricular Flutter

250-350/ min.

In *ventricular flutter,* undulating waves are seen rising and falling. This rhythm is often an intermediary stage between ventricular tachycardia and ventricular fibrillation. The rate is usually between 250 to 350 beats per minute. When the ventricular rate is at this level, the patient is acutely ill and the pulse may be imperceptible. The rate is too fast for ventricular tachycardia, which is usually about 160 beats per minute. This rhythm requires immediate interruption to sustain life. Atrial activity may be unaffected.

Ventricular Fibrillation

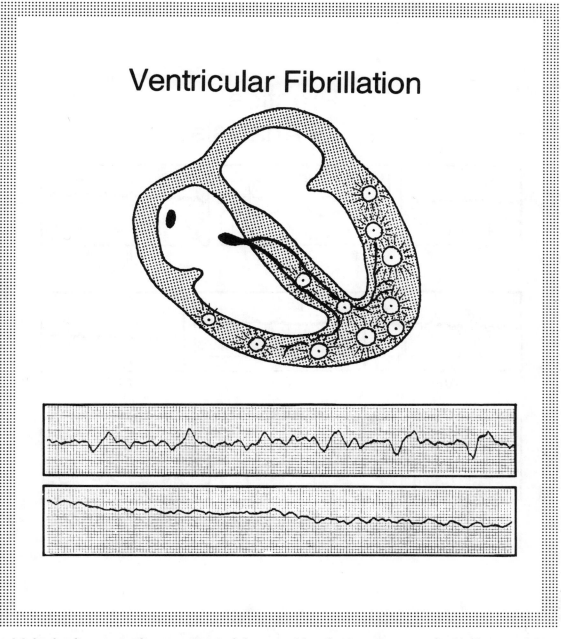

Multiple, disorganized contractions of the ventricles characterize *ventricular fibrillation* and represent *cardiac arrest*. It may be of sudden onset or may follow ventricular premature contractions, ventricular tachycardia and ventricular flutter. The immediate institution of cardiopulmonary resuscitation while waiting for electrical defibrillation may save the patient.

Practice
ECG Analysis

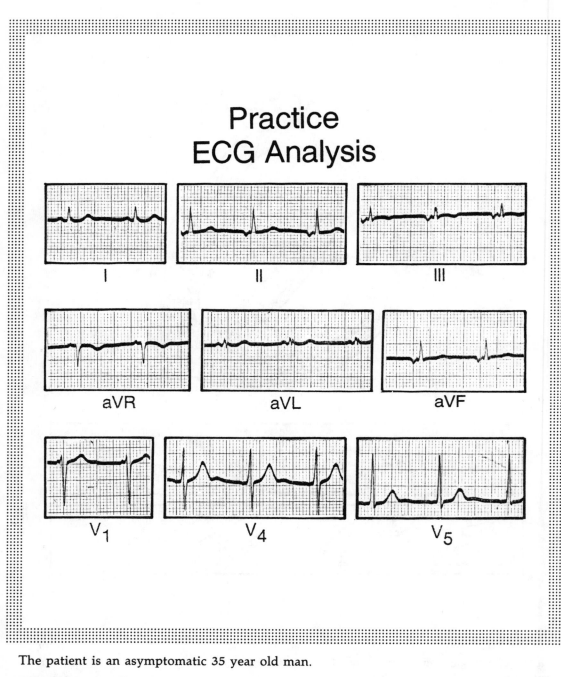

The patient is an asymptomatic 35 year old man.

Analysis:

ECG ANALYSIS

1. Rhythm and Rate
   Rhythm: AV Junctional
   Rate: 85/min.
   PR Interval: 0.1 sec.
   P waves are negative in leads II, III and aVF
2. QRS Complex
   Duration: 0.08 sec.
   Axis: +60°
3. Ventricular Repolarization
   ST Segment: Neither significantly elevated nor depressed
   T wave: QRS-T angle normal
4. QT Interval: 0.35 sec.

Impression and Comment

AV Junctional Rhythm

The AV junction may be the dominant pacemaker congenitally or may share dominance with the SA node throughout life. Since the intrinsic AV junctional rate is 40 to 60 per minute, a rate of 85 per minute is really an AV junctional tachycardia. Many clinicians, however, will not label a rhythm a tachycardia unless the rate is greater than 100 per minute. In an AV junctional rhythm the P waves are usually upright in lead I but may be transitional or slightly negative and negative in leads II and III; they may come before, during or after the QRS complex. When the P wave precedes the QRS complex, the PR interval is usually short, up to 0.12 second. If the atria are not depolarized, a P wave will not be present. The QRS complexes are generally normal, since ventricular depolarization proceeds normally.

Practice
ECG Analysis

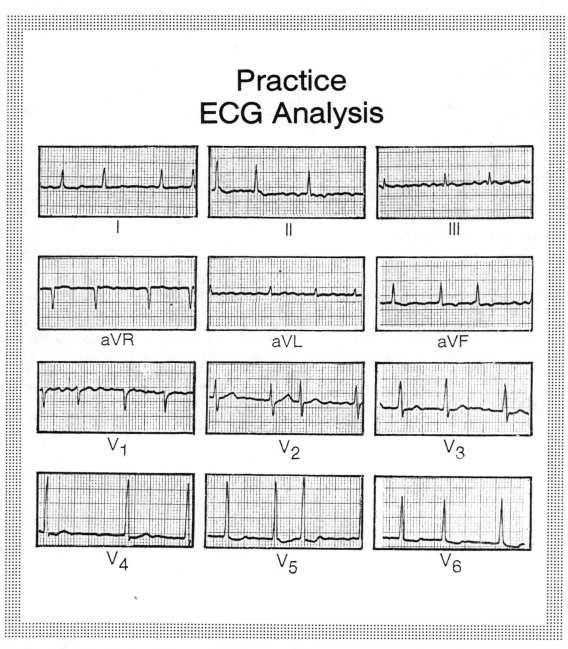

The patient is a 78 year old man with shortness of breath and angina pectoris who discontinued his digitalis one week earlier.

Analysis:

ECG ANALYSIS

1. Rhythm and Rate
   Rhythm: Atrial Fibrillation
   Rate: 95/min., average
   No P waves are present, only fibrillatory atrial waves.
2. QRS Complex
   Duration: 0.08 sec.
   Axis: +45°
3. Ventricular Repolarization
   ST Segment: Depressed, leads II, aVF, V_5, V_6
   T Wave: Low throughout, with a wide QRS-T angle.
4. QT Interval: 0.29 sec.

Impression and Comment

Atrial Fibrillation with Rapid Ventricular Response
Ventricular Repolarization (ST-T) Abnormalities

We see the typical irregularly irregular ventricular response that usually accompanies atrial fibrillation. The ventricular rate depends on how many of 350 to 600 atrial impulses are conducted to the ventricles. One of the actions of digitalis is to increase the block at the AV node, thereby slowing the ventricular rate. Although the patient had not been taking digitalis for one week some "digitalis effects" may still be observed with the rounding of the ST segment depression, best seen in lead V_5. The ST-T abnormalities may be caused predominantly by the myocardial ischemia associated with the patient's coronary heart disease.

Practice
ECG Analysis

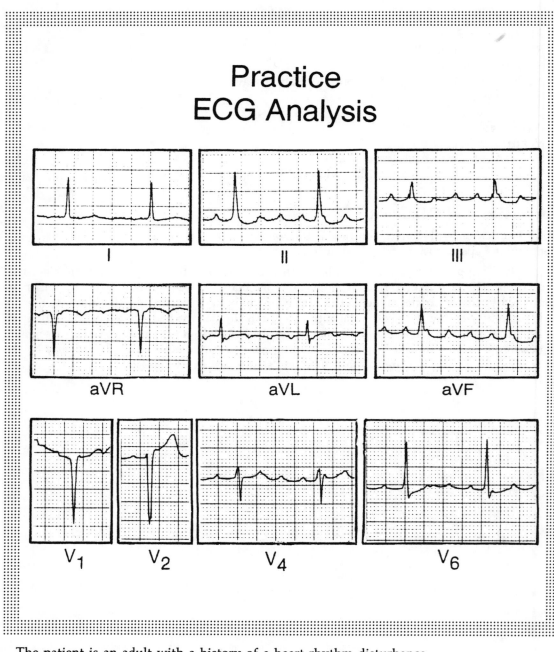

The patient is an adult with a history of a heart rhythm disturbance.

Analysis:

ECG ANALYSIS

1. Rhythm and Rate
   Rhythm: Atrial Flutter with 4:1 AV Block
   Rate: Atrial, 260/min.
   Ventricular, 65/min.
2. QRS Complex
   Duration: 0.08 sec.
   Axis: +45°
3. Ventricular Repolarization
   ST Segment: Depressed and rounded, seen best in leads II, III and aVF.
   T Wave: Difficult to evaluate in the presence of the flutter waves but appears abnormally flat in leads I and V_6
4. QT Interval: 0.36 sec.

Impression and Comment

Atrial Flutter with 4:1 AV Block

Ventricular Repolarization (ST-T) Abnormalities (compatible with digitalis effects and/or ischemia)

With a stable 4:1 relationship between the atria and the ventricles, the ventricular rate is regular at 65 per minute, while the atria are fluttering at a rate of 260 per minute. The rounding of the ST segment suggests that digitalis has been used to treat this patient.

Additional Electrocardiograms for Practice and Review

Practice
ECG Analysis

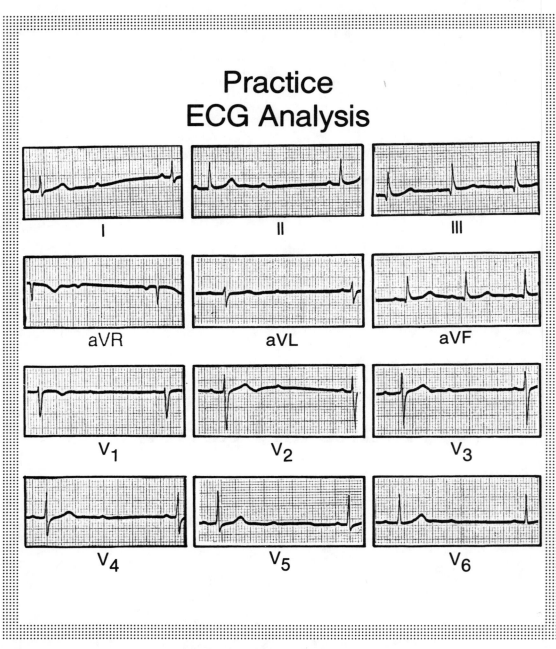

The patient is a 68 year old woman with a complaint of intermittent dizziness.

Analysis:

ECG ANALYSIS

1. Rhythm and Rate
   Rhythm: Second Degree AV Block with 2:1 AV Conduction (except leads III and aVF, where there is 1:1 conduction)
   Rate: Atrial, 68/min.
       Ventricular, 34/min.
   Varying PR intervals, 0.16 sec. to 0.20 sec. (conducted beats)
2. QRS Complex
   Duration: 0.08 sec.
   Axis: + 75°
3. Ventricular Repolarization
   ST Segment: Normal, neither significantly elevated nor depressed
   T Wave: QRS-T angle normal
4. QT Interval: 0.4 sec.

Impression and Comment

Second Degree (2:1) AV Block

The patient had intermittent second degree AV block with a ventricular rate of 34 per minute which was not sufficient to sustain her comfortably. The conducted beats reveal considerable variation in PR intervals, providing a clue as to the problem even when her AV conduction is 1:1. Pacemaker therapy gave her complete relief of symptoms.

Practice
ECG Analysis

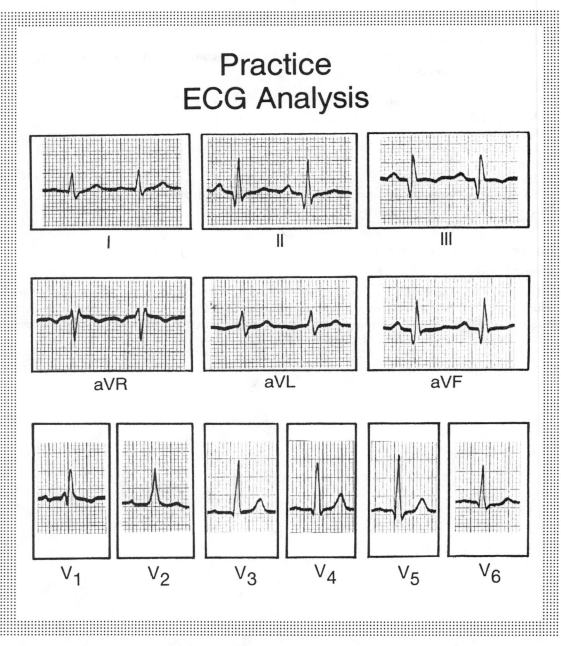

The patient is a 65 year old man with a history of a heart attack 12 years earlier.

Analysis:

ECG ANALYSIS

1. Rhythm and Rate
   Rhythm: Series Rhythm
   Rate: 85/min.
   PR Interval: 0.2 sec.
2. QRS Complex
   Duration: 0.12 sec.
   Axis: +55°
   QRS complex wide, with an S wave in lead I and an R' in lead V_1.
   Significant Q waves in leads II, III and aVF.
3. Ventricular Repolarization
   ST Segment: Neither significantly elevated nor depressed
   T Wave: QRS-T angle normal
4. QT Interval: 0.36 sec.

Impression and Comment

Inferior (Diaphragmatic) Myocardial Infarction; old
Right Bundle Branch Block

The significant Q waves in leads II, III and aVF indicate the inferior (diaphragmatic) my-ocardial infarction. In right bundle branch block the QRS complex is prolonged because of the intraventricular conduction delay. This delay in conduction affects only the *terminal* QRS vector, which is oriented to the *right,* inscribing the S wave in lead I. This terminal QRS vector is also anterior, producing an R' in lead V_1. The *initial* QRS vector is *not* affected by right bundle branch block. The Q waves of myocardial infarction are, therefore, not obscured.

Practice
ECG Analysis

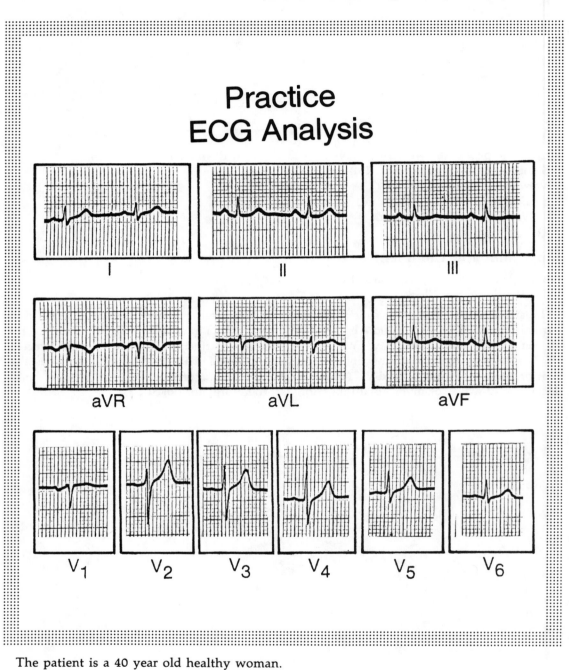

The patient is a 40 year old healthy woman.

Analysis:

ECG ANALYSIS

1. Rhythm and Rate
   Rhythm: Sinus Rhythm
   Rate: 75/min.
   PR Interval: 0.16 sec.
2. QRS Complex
   Duration: 0.08 sec.
   Axis: 75°
3. Ventricular Repolarization
   ST Segment: Neither significantly elevated nor depressed
   T wave: QRS-T angle normal
4. QT Interval: 0.35 sec.

Impression and Comment

Normal Electrocardiogram

Practice
ECG Analysis

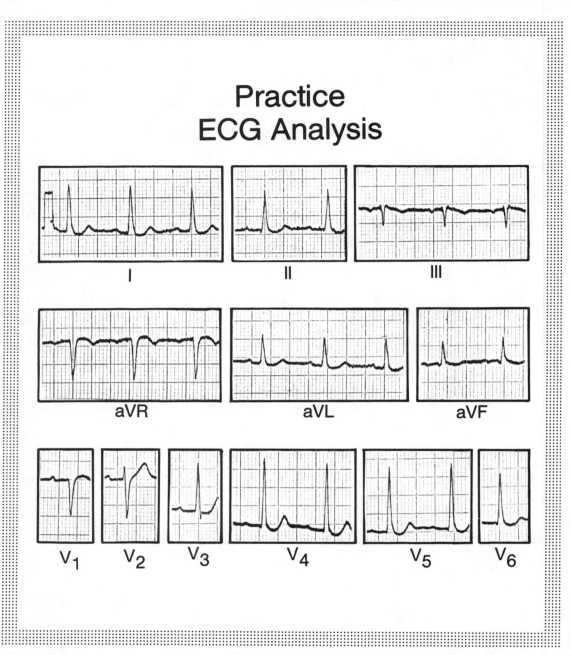

The patient is a 68 year old man with long-standing congestive heart failure. He is taking digitalis and diuretics.

Analysis:

ECG ANALYSIS

1. Rhythm and Rate
   Rhythm: Sinus Rhythm
   Rate: 90/min.
   PR Interval: 0.15 sec.
2. QRS Complex
   Duration: 0.08 sec.
   Axis: + 15°
3. Ventricular Repolarization
   ST Segment: "Paintbrush" inscription in leads I, II, aVL, V_4, V_5 and V_6
   T Wave: QRS-T angle normal
4. QT Interval: 0.32 sec.

Impression and Comment

Ventricular Repolarization Alterations with "Digitalis Effects" on the ST Segment

The classic changes of the ST segment caused by digitalis have been described as a "paint-brush" inscription, as if you were painting the ST segment, with gradual widening of the paintbrush stroke. These changes have also been described as a "fist-like" depression of the ST segment, as if you were placing a fist on the ST segment and depressing it. All of these changes took place when the patient was started on digitalis.

Practice
ECG Analysis

The patient is an 80 year old man with congestive heart failure. He is taking digitalis and diuretics.

Analysis:

ECG ANALYSIS

1. Rhythm and Rate
   Rhythm: Sinus Rhythm
   Rate: 90/min.
   PR Interval: 0.18 sec.
2. QRS Complex
   Duration: 0.16 sec.
   Axis: + 15°
   QS complexes in leads V_1 and V_2
   Absence of the small normal Q waves in leads I, aVL, V_5 and V_6
3. Ventricular Repolarization
   ST Segment: Depressed in leads I, II, aVF, V_5 and V_6
   T Wave: Inverted in leads I, II, V_5 and V_6, wide QRS-T angle
4. QT Interval: 0.35 sec.

Impression and Comment

Left Bundle Branch Block.

Review the criteria for left bundle branch block. All are present here.
   1. The QRS interval is 0.16 sec.
   2. QS complexes in leads V_1 and V_2
   3. Absence of small normal Q waves in leads I, aVL, V_5 and V_6
   4. Marked repolarization abnormalities

The QS complexes in leads V_1 and V_2 are the result of the left bundle branch and should *not* be interpreted as anterior or anteroseptal myocardial infarction. Left bundle branch block may simulate or mask myocardial infarction.

Practice
ECG Analysis

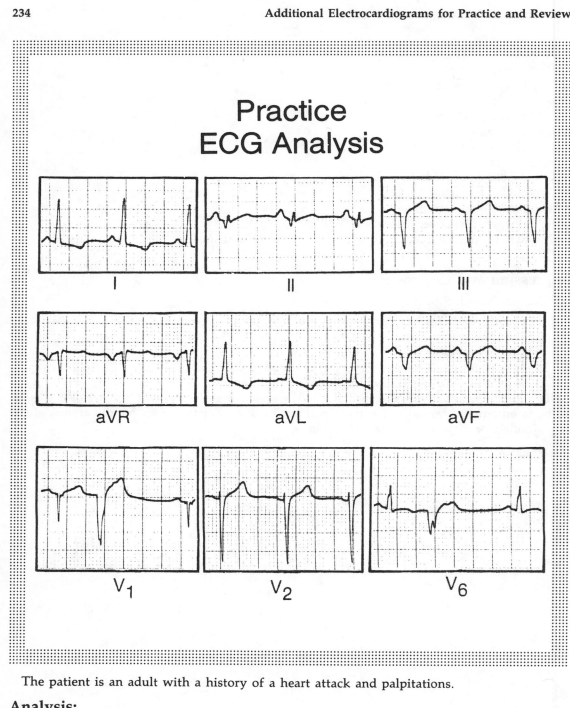

The patient is an adult with a history of a heart attack and palpitations.

Analysis:

ECG ANALYSIS

1. Rhythm and Rate
   Rhythm: Sinus Rhythm
   Rate: 85/min.
   PR Interval: 0.14 sec.
2. QRS Complex
   Duration: 0.08 sec.
   Axis: $-25°$
   Significant Q waves in leads II, III and aVF
   Premature ventricular contractions in leads V_1 and V_6.
3. Ventricular Repolarization
   ST Segment: Depressed in leads I and aVL
   T Wave: Inverted in leads I, aVL and V_6, wide QRS-T angle.
4. QT Interval: 0.35 sec.

Impression and Comment

Inferior (Diaphragmatic) Myocardial Infarction, Old
Left Axis Deviation
Ventricular Repolarization (ST-T) Abnormalities
Premature Ventricular Contractions

There is electrocardiographic evidence of ischemia (ST-T abnormalities) and irritability (premature ventricular contractions) in addition to the old infarction. Careful evaluation is required in view of the already compromised coronary circulation.

Practice
ECG Analysis

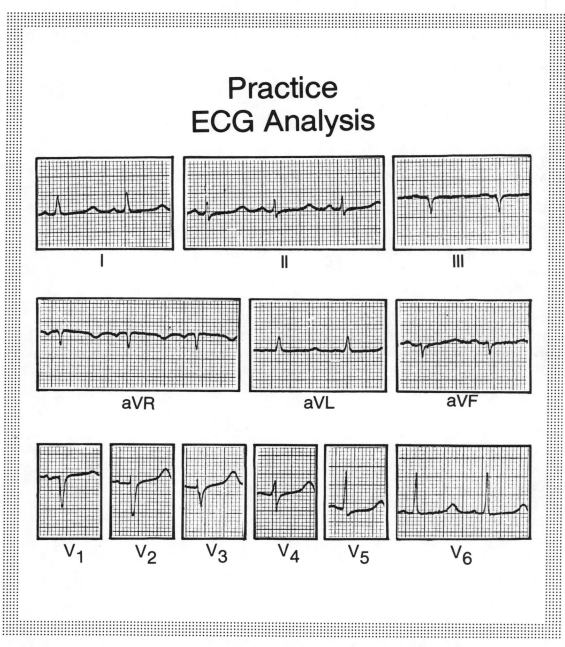

The patient is a 75 year old woman with a long history of hypoparathyroidism.

Analysis:

ECG ANALYSIS

1. Rhythm and Rate
   Rhythm: Sinus Rhythm
   Rate: 80/min.
   PR Interval: 0.14 sec.
2. QRS Complex
   Duration: 0.08 sec.
   Axis: −15°
3. Ventricular Repolarization
   ST Segment: neither significantly elevated nor depressed
   T Wave: Normal QRS-T angle.
4. QT Interval: 0.52 sec.

Impression and Comment

QT Interval Markedly Prolonged, Compatible with Hypocalcemia

Marked prolongation of the QT interval is compatible with the hypocalcemia of hypoparathyroidism. At this patient's heart rate of 84 per minute, the QT interval should be approximately 0.35 second, rather than 0.52 second, as seen here. The relationship between the QT interval and the heart rate is as follows:

Heart Rate/min	QT Interval (sec.)
40	0.46
60	0.39
80	0.35
100	0.31
120	0.29
140	0.26
160	0.25

Practice
ECG Analysis

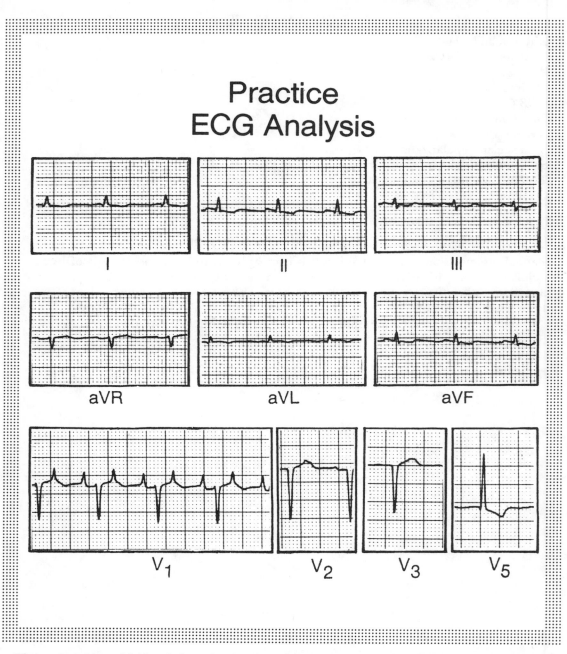

The patient is an elderly adult with a history of a heart attack and a heart rhythm disturbance.

Analysis:

ECG ANALYSIS

1. Rhythm and Rate
   Rhythm: Atrial Tachycardia with 2:1 AV Block
   Rate: Atrial, 188/min.
         Ventricular, 94/min.
   PR Interval: 0.15 sec.
2. QRS Complex
   Duration: 0.08 sec.
   Axis: +30°
   Significant Q waves seen best in leads V_2 and V_3
3. Ventricular Repolarization
   ST Segment: Depressed in leads I, II, and V_5
   T Wave: Wide QRS-T angle
4. QT Interval: 0.32 sec.

Impression and Comment

Anteroseptal Myocardial Infarction, Old
Atrial Tachycardia with 2:1 AV Block
Ventricular Repolarization (ST-T) Abnormalities

The findings on this electrocardiogram emphasize the need to examine the entire electro-cardiogram. Without the precordial leads, it would be impossible to come to the above con-clusions. Although the frontal plane leads (I, II, III, aVR, aVL, and aVF) reveal an abnormal electrocardiogram with ST-T abnormalities, the precordial leads in the horizontal plane reveal both the arrhythmia and the old myocardial infarction. If the atrial rate were faster (250 to 350 per minute), atrial flutter would be considered.

Practice
ECG Analysis

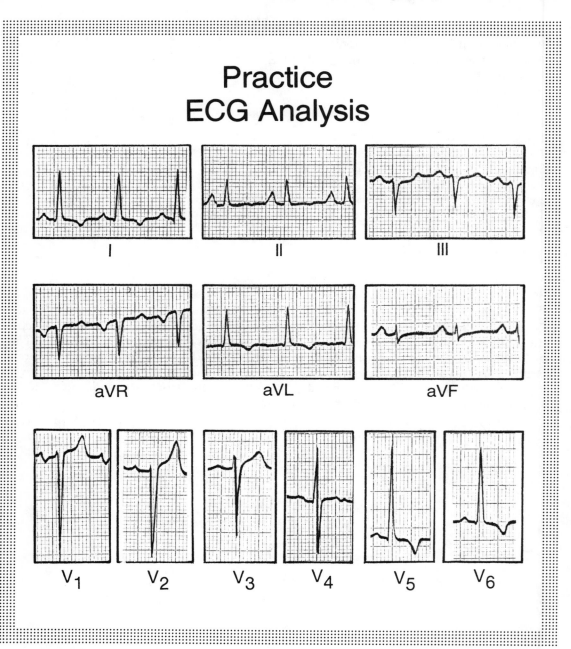

The patient is a 78 year old man with a long history of hypertension and congestive heart failure. Blood pressure at present is 130/80 mm. Hg. His medication includes digitalis and diuretics.

Analysis:

ECG ANALYSIS

1. Rhythm and Rate
   Rhythm: Sinus Rhythm
   Rate: 92/min.
   PR Interval: 0.18 sec.
   Tall, peaked P waves, leads II and aVF
   Diphasic P waves, lead V_1, overall size, 3 mm.
2. QRS Complex
   Duration: 0.09 sec.
   Axis: 0°
   $S_{V_1} + R_{V_5} = 55$ mm.
3. Ventricular Repolarization
   ST Segment: Neither significantly elevated nor depressed
   T Wave: very wide QRS-T angle.
4. QT Interval: 0.32 sec.

Impression and Comment

Right Atrial and Ventricular Hypertrophy
Left Atrial and Ventricular Hypertrophy
Ventricular Repolarization Abnormalities

Right atrial hypertrophy is reflected in the tall, peaked P waves, seen especially well in lead II. Right atrial hypertrophy is good *presumptive* evidence of right ventricular hypertrophy, since it rarely occurs without right ventricular hypertrophy. Direct electrocardiographic evidence of right ventricular hypertrophy is often obscured by the dominant left ventricle.

Left atrial hypertrophy is best seen in lead V_1. The normal P wave in lead V_1 is usually 1 to 2 mm. Here we have a P wave of 3 mm., with the second half of the diphasic P wave significantly negative. The criteria for left ventricular hypertrophy include the great magnitude of the QRS complexes in addition to the associated repolarization abnormalities.

This elderly patient had a very large heart and hypertrophy of all four chambers.

Practice
ECG Analysis

I	II	III

aVR	aVL	aVF

V$_1$	V$_2$	V$_3$	V$_4$	V$_5$	V$_6$

The patient is a 78 year old man who had a heart attack 10 years earlier. He suffers from chronic congestive heart failure.

Analysis:

ECG ANALYSIS

1. Rhythm and Rate
   Rhythm: AV Junctional
   Rate: 62/min.
   PR Interval: 0.11 sec.
   P waves are positive in lead I and negative in leads II, III, and aVF.
2. QRS Complex
   Duration: 0.11 sec.
   Axis: $-45°$
   Broad Q waves, best in V_2 to V_5
   The QRS complex in lead V_1 is 30 mm. in size
3. Ventricular Repolarization
   ST Segment: Elevated and rounded with a "curve of injury" pattern in leads V_1 to V_5
   T Wave: Inverted in leads I, aVL, V_4 to V_5 and flat in V_6, where normally they are upright
4. QT Interval: 0.4 sec.

Impression and Comment

AV Junctional Rhythm
Left Axis Deviation
Ventricular Aneurysm
Anterior Myocardial Infarction, Old
Left Ventricular Hypertrophy
Ventricular Repolarization (ST-T) Abnormalities
QRS Interval Prolonged

The P waves are positive in lead I and negative in leads II, III and aVF, resulting in a left axis deviation of the mean P vector. The latter, together with the short PR interval, reveal the AV junctional rhythm. The elevated and rounded ST segments with a "curve of injury" pattern resembling the evolutionary changes of an acute myocardial infarction represent the ventricular aneurysm. The broad, slurred Q waves, seen especially well in leads V_2 to V_5, reflect the anterior myocardial infarction sustained 10 years earlier. The large size of the QRS complexes, especially lead V_1, of more than 30 mm. signifies left ventricular hypertrophy. The marked ventricular repolarization (ST-T) abnormalities are compatible with the patient's known myocardial ischemia. The prolongation of the QRS interval reveals an intraventricular conduction delay.

Practice
ECG Analysis

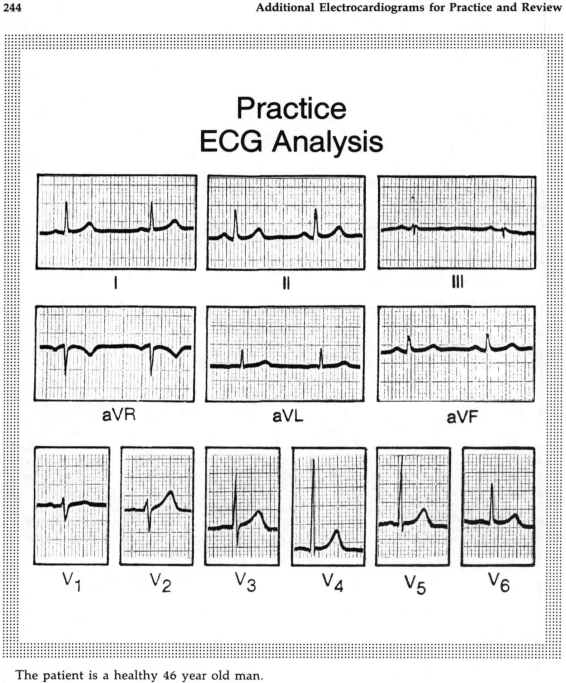

The patient is a healthy 46 year old man.

Analysis:

ECG ANALYSIS

1. Rhythm and Rate
   Rhythm: Sinus Rhythm
   Rate: 67/min.
   PR Interval: 0.14 sec.
2. QRS Complex
   Duration: 0.08 sec.
   Axis: 30°
3. Ventricular Repolarization
   ST Segment: Neither significantly elevated nor depressed.
   T Wave: QRS-T angle normal
4. QT Interval: 0.36 sec.

Impression and Comment

Normal Electrocardiogram

Practice
ECG Analysis

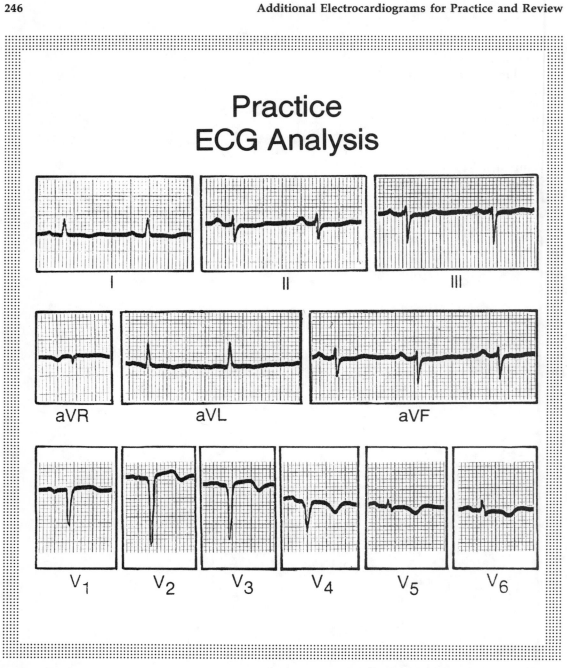

The patient is a 59 year old man recuperating from a heart attack suffered one month earlier.

Analysis:

ECG ANALYSIS

1. Rhythm and Rate
   Rhythm: Sinus Rhythm
   Rate: 67/min.
   PR Interval: 0.2 sec.
2. QRS Complex
   Duration: 0.09 sec.
   Axis: $-45°$
   QS complexes, leads V_1 to V_4
3. Ventricular Repolarization
   ST Segment: Elevated, especially leads V_2 and V_3
   T Wave: Wide QRS-T angle
4. QT Interval: 0.4 sec.

Impression and Comment

Anterior Myocardial Infarction, Evolving
Left Axis Deviation
Ventricular Repolarization (ST-T) Abnormalities

Since we do not have an electrocardiogram taken prior to the myocardial infarction, we are unable to determine whether the left axis deviation or the wide QRS-T angle is the result of the myocardial infarction or was present before. The elevated ST segments reflect the evolving changes occurring as a result of a recent myocardial infarction.

Index